Making Sense of VA Disability

VETERAN ROLLCALL

A Veteran's Guide to Ratings, Compensation & Appeals

J. Wiltz Cutrer, Jr.

Making Sense of VA Disability

Veteran Roll Call Series, Book Two

Please make direct requests for permission to make copies of any part of this work or to request the author speak at your event to:

wiltz@VeteranRollCall.org

Visit us on the web:

VeteranRollCall.org

Cover Design: *Brian Kittrell*

ISBN: 978-0-9885928-5-8

Library of Congress Control Number: 2026906963

First Edition | 2026

Part of the Veteran Roll Call Series, a collection of plain-language guides designed to help Veterans and families navigate Department of Veterans Affairs benefits with clarity and confidence.

Printed in the United States of America

Published by TechKnolutions, LLC, Brandon, MS

Dedication

Families shape us in ways nothing else can. They steady us, challenge us, and remind us of who we are when life gets loud. Mine has done all of that and more, guiding me with love, patience, and the kind of honesty only family can give. They are my compass, my reminder of what truly matters, and the greatest blessings God could have trusted me with.

Kristen, Wiltz III, and Izzy

To my wife, Kristen — thank you for walking beside me through every step of my own VA journey, long before this book ever existed. Your support has been steady, patient, and unwavering... even on the days when I was less than easy to support. Your strength has carried me farther than you know.

To my son, Wiltz III — you continue to inspire me every single day. Your kindness, drive, and quiet confidence remind me of the best parts of life. Stay true to yourself, always. The world needs exactly who you are — even if you occasionally roll your eyes at your old man.

To my daughter, Izzy — you have a gift for keeping me honest, sharpening my thinking, and challenging me in ways that make me better. Your curiosity and quick wit pushes me to grow, even when I didn't know I needed the nudge

I am proud of each of you — deeply and humbly proud. Thank you for being my foundation, my joy, and the reminder that family is where our greatest strength is found.

The Veteran Roll Call Series

This series was created with one mission in mind: to give Veterans and their families clear, trustworthy guidance through the complex world of Department of Veterans Affairs benefits. Every book is written in plain language, grounded in real experience, and focused on helping you understand what you've earned — and how to access it with confidence. No jargon. No government-speak. No need for a pot of coffee strong enough to power a destroyer.

In the first book, *Making Sense of What You've Earned: A Veteran's Guide to Benefits and Resources*, we provide a broad foundation across the full range of VA programs — disability compensation, pension, education, housing, health care, mental health services, and family support. It's designed to help you see the entire landscape of benefits available to you, all in one place.

This book builds on that foundation by taking a deeper, more focused look at VA disability — how ratings work, how claims are evaluated, what evidence matters, and how to navigate exams, secondary conditions, and appeals. It stands fully on its own, but readers of the first book will recognize the same step-by-step approach, practical tools, and myth-busting clarity.

Future books will continue this mission with dedicated guides on VA health care, mental health resources, caregiver support, and more. Together, these books form a complete, accessible roadmap for Veterans and families who want to understand their benefits — not just in theory, but in practice.

Knowledge is power. Clarity is freedom.

You served. You earned these benefits.

This series helps you make sense of them.

Other Books in This Series

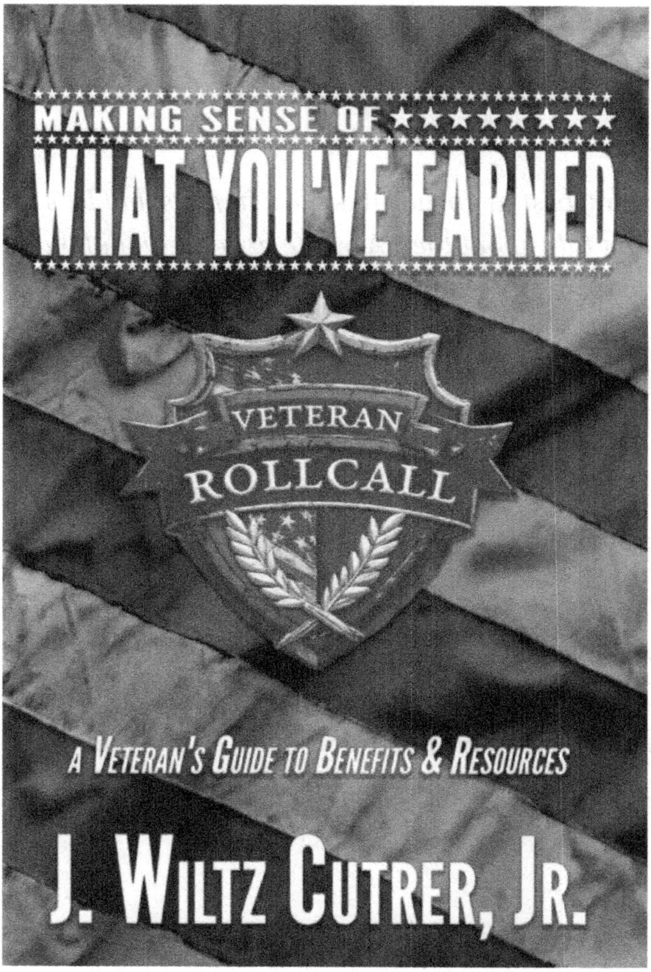

Veteran benefits don't have to be confusing. This empowering guide cuts through myths, acronyms, and red tape to show veterans and families exactly what they've earned—and how to claim it. Clear, practical, and compassionate, it transforms frustration into confidence and makes the VA system finally approachable.

You served. You earned these benefits.
Now it's time to use them.

† † † † †

I've done my best to anchor this book in facts, but let's be real — you can't talk about the VA or life in general without a little perspective mixed in. Some readers may see a solution here and think, "I'd handle that differently." And that's perfectly fine. Different experiences lead to different viewpoints, and that's what keeps things interesting.

The opinions and approaches I share come from my journey, just as yours come from yours.

And for the record: I haven't received any compensation, sponsorships, or behind-the-scenes perks from any company or organization mentioned. No endorsements, no incentives — just my honest experiences, shared in the hope they make your path a bit smoother.

† † † † †

Table of Contents

COMMON PITFALL:

Assuming you'll "remember everything later."
Keep a simple symptom journal —
even a few notes each month can help
if you ever need an increase or appeal.

† † † † †

COMMON PITFALL:

Thinking you have to "figure it all out"
before you start.
You don't.
You just need a guide — and now you have one.

† † † † †

PROLOGUE

If you're holding this book, chances are you've already discovered something important about the VA benefits system: it's not exactly a "*grab a cup of coffee and breeze through it*" kind of experience.

In fact, for many Veterans and families, the VA process feels a bit like being handed a 5,000-piece puzzle... without the picture on the box... and with a few pieces that look suspiciously like they belong to someone else's puzzle entirely.

But here's the good news:

You don't have to figure it out alone.

And you definitely don't have to guess.

This book is your map, your flashlight, and your "*hey, don't step in that*" guide to navigating the VA benefits world with clarity, confidence, and maybe even a few laughs along the way.

Because yes — we're going to talk about forms, evidence, claims, appeals, and acronyms that look like someone spilled alphabet soup on a government keyboard. But we're also going to talk about real people. Real families. Real stories. Real victories. And the real impact these benefits can have on a Veteran's life.

You'll learn what works, what doesn't, and why the phrase "*at least as likely as not*" is more powerful than it sounds. You'll see how to avoid the potholes that trip up so many Veterans. You'll understand how to support someone you love through the process. And you'll discover that the VA system — while complicated — is navigable with the right tools.

Most importantly, you'll realize what far too many Veterans forget:

You earned these benefits.

You deserve these benefits.

And you are fully capable of getting them.

This book isn't here to overwhelm you. It's here to empower you. To simplify the complicated. To translate the confusion. To give you the confidence to take the next step — whether you're filing your first claim, helping a family member, or trying to make sense of a decision letter that reads like it was written by a committee of very tired lawyers.

So, take a breath.
Grab a pen.
Maybe grab a snack — *snacks help*.
And let's walk this path together.

Whether this is your first time joining me or you've already read the first book in this series, I'm glad you're here. You've already done the hard part: you showed up. Now let's get you the clarity, support, and benefits you've earned.

Understanding VA Compensation

Understanding how the VA thinks about disability ratings is half the battle. Once you know the rules, the process becomes far less intimidating.

VA compensation is often the first benefit Veterans hear about—and one of the most misunderstood. This chapter breaks down what compensation really is, how the VA decides disability ratings, and what those percentages actually mean in real life. No legal jargon, no guesswork—just a clear, honest explanation of how service-connected disability pay works, why it exists, and how it can support you and your family.

Myth vs. Reality: *VA Compensation*

- **Myth:** "*VA compensation is just the VA being generous.*"

  Reality: VA compensation is not a gift—it's a benefit you earned through service and the impact of your disabilities.

- **Myth:** "*If my buddy has 70% for the same condition, I should too.*"

  Reality: The VA doesn't rate diagnoses; it rates *how much they affect your life*. Two people with the same condition can have very different ratings.

- **Myth:** "*If I can still work, I won't qualify.*"

  Reality: Many Veterans receive compensation and still work. The question is how your conditions limit you—not whether you're employed.

What is VA Disability Compensation?

If you've ever tried to explain the VA disability system to someone who hasn't dealt with it, you've probably seen that familiar expression — the polite nod paired with the quiet panic of someone who suddenly realizes they've stepped into a conversation they weren't prepared for. And honestly, who can blame them? The VA's Compensation and Pension program, or "*C&P*," has a reputation for being complicated, mysterious, and occasionally as clear as a mud puddle after a rainstorm.

But at its core, VA disability compensation is simple. It's the government's way of acknowledging your military service came with a cost — sometimes physical, sometimes mental, sometimes both — and that cost didn't magically disappear when you turned in your gear. The monthly payment you receive is tax-free and meant to help offset the impact of those service-connected conditions on your daily life.

Eligibility is more straightforward than most people expect. You generally need three things:

- A current disability or condition
- A connection between that condition and your military service
- A discharge that isn't dishonorable

That's it. No secret handshake, no hidden password, no need to sacrifice a Humvee to the VA gods (*though many have tried*). The purpose of the program is to compensate you for the ways your service-connected conditions affect your ability to function and earn a living. It's not a reward. It's not charity. It's earned — plain and simple.

Here's the heart of it: if your time in uniform left you with hearing loss, a back that sounds like a bowl of Rice Krispies, migraines that show up uninvited, or any number of other issues, the VA's job is to evaluate those conditions and assign a rating that reflects their severity. That rating becomes the foundation for your monthly compensation.

How Ratings Work

Now we get to the part of the VA system that has confused more Veterans than the phrase "*hurry up and wait.*" Disability ratings come from something called the VA Schedule for Rating Disabilities – the VASRD. Despite the intimidating name, it's really just a massive rulebook that lists medical conditions and explains how the VA evaluates them.

Each condition has its own criteria. The VA looks at how much that condition affects your ability to function and assigns a percentage rating. These ratings run from 0 percent to 100 percent in steps of ten. A 0 percent rating means the condition is service-connected but doesn't currently impact your earning ability. A 100 percent rating means the condition is totally disabling.

To make this feel less abstract, imagine you have chronic knee pain. The VASRD has a section specifically for knee conditions. It looks at things like range of motion, instability, pain levels, and how the knee affects your ability to walk or stand. Based on those factors, the VA assigns a percentage. It's not random – it's tied to the criteria in the schedule.

Where things get interesting – and by "*interesting,*" I mean "*mathematically creative*" – is when you have more than one disability. Most people assume the VA simply adds the percentages together like a whole number. For example, 50 percent plus 30 percent would equal 80 percent. But you must remember, these are percentages and <u>not</u> whole numbers (*and it is not common core math, either*).

Instead, the VA uses what's often called "*VA math.*" The idea is that your body starts at 100 percent efficiency. Each disability reduces that efficiency, but the reduction applies to whatever efficiency remains. Think of it like taking slices out of a pie – each slice is taken from what's left, <u>not</u> from the original whole.

Here's a simple visual to show how it works:

Start:
100% efficient

↓ minus 50% disability

50% remaining

↓ minus 30% of remaining 50% (15%)

Final = 65% → rounded to 70%

Once you see it laid out, the logic becomes clearer. The VA isn't adding percentages; it's subtracting from what's left of your "*healthy*" efficiency.

Example 2:
Two Disabilities

Let's say you have:

- 50 percent for PTSD
- 30 percent for your knee

Here's how the VA calculates it:

Start: 100% efficient – Apply 50% disability:

100% - 50% = 50% remaining

Apply 30% disability:

30% of 50% = 15%

50 + 15 = 65%

Final combined rating = 65% → rounded to 70%

So instead of 80 percent, you end up at 70 percent. This surprises a lot of Veterans the first time they see it, but once you understand the pattern, it starts to make sense.

Example 3:
Three Disabilities

Now let's look at a slightly more realistic scenario. You have:

- 40 percent for your back
- 20 percent for your knee
- 10 percent for tinnitus

Here's the math:

Start: 100% efficient – Apply 40% disability:

100% - 40% = 60% remaining

<u>Apply 20% disability:</u>

20% of 60% = 12%

40 + 12 = 52%

<u>Apply 10% disability:</u>

10% of 52% = 5.2%

40 + 12 + 5.2 = 57.2%

Final combined rating = 57.2% → rounded to 60%

So even though the individual ratings may "*appear*" to add up to a higher number, the combined rating becomes 60 percent. This is why understanding VA math early on is so important — it helps set expectations and prevents a lot of frustration later.

Why the VA Does It This Way

The VA's logic is that each disability affects whatever "*healthy*" part of you remains. Whether you agree with that logic is a separate conversation, but the system is consistent. Once you understand the pattern, you can predict your combined rating with surprising accuracy.

Later chapters will walk you through more examples, including bilateral factors, special situations, and how to estimate your rating before you file a claim.

Understanding how the VA calculates your combined disability rating is a big step, and if you've made it this far without needing a cup of coffee or a quiet moment to stare out a window, you're already ahead of the game. VA math may not be intuitive, but once you see how the pieces fit together, the system starts to feel a lot less mysterious.

Now that you know how the VA arrives at your final rating, in the next section, we'll break down how the VA turns that rating into a tax-free monthly payment — and how your family situation can affect the final amount

---

† † † † †

Most Veterans underestimate their symptoms
because they've learned to "push through."
The VA can't rate what you don't report.

† † † † †

Monthly Payment Basics

Once your disability ratings are established, the next natural question is, "*Alright, so what does that mean for my monthly check?*" This is the moment where most Veterans lean in a little closer, because the rating is important — but the payment is what actually shows up in your bank account.

VA disability compensation is tax-free and based on three main ingredients:

- Your combined disability rating
- Your dependency status (*spouse, children, dependent parents*)
- Whether you qualify for any additional special monthly compensation

The VA updates the payment tables every year, usually in line with the Social Security cost-of-living adjustment. That means your payment can increase slightly each year to keep up with inflation. You don't have to apply for this increase — it happens automatically.

Why Dependents Affect Your Payment

Many Veterans are surprised to learn that the VA pays more if you have dependents. The logic is simple: supporting a family costs money, and disabilities can make that harder. If you're rated 30 percent or higher, the VA adds extra compensation for:

- A spouse
- Children under 18
- Children between 18 and 23 who are in school
- Dependent parents

This isn't meant to cover every expense of raising a family, but it does help offset the added financial responsibilities.

A Simple Example:

Let's say you're rated at 70 percent. The VA's compensation table lists a base amount for a single Veteran at 70 percent. If you have a spouse, that amount increases. Add a child, and it increases again. Add a second child, and so on.

Here's a simplified illustration of how it works conceptually:

Base rate for 70% rating

+ amount for spouse

+ amount for first child

+ amount for additional children (*if any*)

= your total monthly payment

If that same Veteran later gets married, the payment increases again. If a child turns 18 and is not in school, the payment decreases. The system is designed to adjust as your life changes.

You don't need to memorize the numbers — the VA publishes the exact amounts each year. What matters is understanding that your payment adjusts to reflect your family situation.

---

† † † † †

COMMON PITFALL:

Focusing only on the diagnosis and forgetting to describe how the condition affects daily life. Functionality is the key to accurate ratings.

† † † † †

What You Don't Need to Worry About

You don't need to calculate your payment by hand. You don't need to guess. And you definitely don't need to keep a spreadsheet unless you just enjoy spreadsheets. The VA's tables do the heavy lifting. Your job is simply to understand the moving parts, so the numbers make sense when you see them.

The goal of the compensation program is to provide financial support that reflects both the severity of your service-connected conditions and the realities of your life. It's not meant to make you wealthy, but it is meant to help you live with stability, dignity, and a little less financial pressure

---

By now, you've seen how the VA determines whether a condition is service-connected, how the rating system works (*including the infamous VA math*), and how those ratings translate into monthly compensation. You've taken the first big step toward understanding a system that often feels more complicated than it needs to be, and you've done it without needing a law degree, a calculator, or a stiff drink. That's a win in my book.

But Compensation is only one side of the VA's financial support programs. There's another benefit — one that's often misunderstood, sometimes overlooked, and occasionally confused with Compensation even though it works very differently. It's called VA Pension, and it serves a completely different purpose. In the next chapter, we'll break down what Pension is, who qualifies, how it's calculated, and how to know whether Pension or Compensation is the right path for your situation. Think of Chapter 2 as the companion piece to everything you've just learned — same VA, different mission.

Understanding VA Pension

Surviving spouses may qualify for the pension even if the Veteran never filed a claim during their lifetime.

VA pension is one of the most powerful yet overlooked benefits available to wartime Veterans and their families. Many people assume it's only for those with no income at all—but the truth is more nuanced and often more generous. In this chapter, we'll unpack who qualifies, how income and medical expenses are counted, and how pension can provide critical support in later life or during times of financial strain.

Myth vs. Reality: *VA Pension*

- **Myth:** "*VA pension is only for Veterans with no income at all.*"

  Reality: Pension is based on **net** income after medical expenses. Many Veterans qualify once their care costs are counted.

- **Myth:** "*You have to have been in combat to get pension.*"

  Reality: You only need **wartime service**, not combat. Serving during a qualifying period is what matters.

- **Myth:** "*If the Veteran never filed a claim, the surviving spouse is out of luck.*"

  Reality: Surviving spouses may still qualify for pension or other benefits—even if the Veteran never filed during their lifetime.

What is VA Pension?

If Chapter 1 was all about VA Compensation — the benefit tied to disabilities caused or worsened by military service — then VA Pension is its quieter, often misunderstood cousin. Many Veterans have heard of it, some confuse it with Compensation, and a few assume it's something you only get if you've retired from the military. None of those assumptions are quite right.

VA Pension is a needs-based financial benefit for wartime Veterans who have limited income and meet certain age or disability requirements. Think of it as the VA's safety net — a program designed to help Veterans who served during a period of war but now face financial hardship later in life.

The biggest difference between Pension and Compensation is simple:

- Compensation is about service-connected disabilities.
- Pension is about financial need.

You could have no service-connected disabilities at all and still qualify for Pension if your income is low enough and you meet the other criteria. On the flip side, you could have multiple disabilities from service and still not qualify for Pension if your income is above the threshold. The two programs serve different missions, even though they both come from the VA and both provide monthly payments.

Here's a helpful way to think about it:

- Compensation asks: "*Did your military service cause or worsen a disability?*"
- Pension asks: "*Did you serve during a wartime period, and do you now have limited income or resources?*"

Both programs are tax-free. Both are monthly payments. Both are meant to support Veterans. But they operate on completely different foundations.

Many Veterans don't realize they might qualify for Pension, especially if they never filed for Compensation or don't have service-connected conditions. Others may qualify for both programs but can only receive one at a time — and choosing the right path can make a big difference in long-term financial stability. We'll get into that later in this chapter.

For now, the key takeaway is this: VA Pension exists to help wartime Veterans who need financial support, regardless of whether their health issues are connected to their service. It's a benefit with a very specific purpose and understanding that purpose is the first step in figuring out whether it's the right fit for you or someone you're helping.

Before we go any further, it's important to understand who actually qualifies for VA Pension. Unlike Compensation, which focuses on service-connected disabilities, Pension has its own set of rules — and they're built around wartime service, financial need, and age or disability status. Once you understand these criteria, the rest of the program starts to make a lot more sense. The next section will explore eligibility for the pension benefit.

---

† † † † †

Many Veterans miss out on pensions for years
simply because they didn't know their assisted-living costs
could be deducted.
Don't let that be you.

† † † † †

Eligibility Criteria

If VA Pension had a slogan, it would probably be something like: *"Not everyone qualifies, but if you do, we want you to know."* Pension is one of those benefits that sounds simple on the surface but has a few moving parts underneath. The good news is that once you understand the criteria, the whole picture becomes much clearer.

VA Pension eligibility is built on three pillars: **wartime service**, **limited income**, and **age or disability status**. All three matter, and all three work together.

Wartime Service

This is the first and most fundamental requirement. VA Pension is specifically for Veterans who served during a recognized period of war. You don't have to have been in combat. You don't have to have deployed. You don't even have to have left the continental United States. You simply need to have served at least one day during an official wartime period and meet the minimum active-duty service requirement for your era.

This is where many Veterans are surprised. They'll say, *"But I never went overseas,"* or *"I was stateside the whole time."* That doesn't matter. If your service dates fall within a wartime window, you meet this part of the requirement.

Income and Net Worth Limits

Unlike Compensation, which doesn't care how much money you make, Pension is a needs-based program. That means the VA looks at your household income and net worth to determine whether you qualify.

The VA sets an annual income limit called the Maximum Annual Pension Rate (MAPR). If your countable income is below that limit, you may qualify. If it's above the limit, you may not – though certain medical expenses can be deducted, which can bring your countable income down.

This is where Pension can get a little technical, but the core idea is simple: the program is designed to help wartime Veterans who genuinely need financial support.

Age or Disability Requirements

To qualify for Pension, you must also meet one of the following:

- Be 65 or older,
- Have a permanent and total disability,
- Be a patient in a nursing home due to disability, or
- Be receiving Social Security Disability Insurance (SSDI) or Supplemental Security Income (SSI).

This is another area where Veterans sometimes misunderstand the program. You don't need a service-connected disability to qualify. You don't need a VA rating at all. Pension looks at your overall health and ability to work, not whether your conditions are tied to your military service.

Putting It All Together

To be eligible for VA Pension, you must meet **all** of the following:

- You served during a wartime period
- You meet the income and net worth limits
- You meet the age or disability requirements
- You were discharged under conditions other than dishonorable

If you check all those boxes, you're in the right place. If you're unsure about any of them, don't worry — later sections will walk you through how the VA calculates income, what counts as a deductible expense, and how special circumstances like Aid & Attendance can increase your benefit.

VA Pension may not be as widely understood as Compensation, but for the Veterans who qualify, it can be a vital source of stability and support.

Once you know the basic eligibility requirements for Pension, the next step is understanding how the benefit can expand when a Veteran's needs increase. That's where Special Monthly Pension comes in — additional support for those who require extra help with daily living or who are largely confined to their home. We'll discuss this in our next section.

Special Monthly Pension (*Aid & Attendance, Housebound*)

If VA Pension is the base layer of support, then Special Monthly Pension is the extra help the VA offers when a Veteran's needs go beyond the basics. Think of it as the VA recognizing that sometimes life requires more than just keeping the lights on — sometimes you need assistance with daily activities, or you're limited in how far you can safely move around your home. That's where Aid & Attendance (A&A) and Housebound benefits come in.

These aren't separate programs. They're add-ons to Pension — extra amounts the VA pays when a Veteran's health or living situation requires a higher level of support. You can only receive them if you already qualify for VA Pension, but once you do, these additions can significantly increase your monthly benefit.

Aid & Attendance (A&A)

Aid & Attendance is designed for Veterans who need help with the everyday tasks most people take for granted. This doesn't mean you need full-time nursing care or a medical team following you around. It simply means you require regular assistance to stay safe and maintain your quality of life.

A Veteran may qualify for A&A if they:

- Need help with activities of daily living (*bathing, dressing, eating, toileting, adjusting prosthetics*)
- Are bedridden due to illness
- Live in a nursing home because of physical or mental limitations
- Have eyesight limited to a certain level

The VA isn't looking for perfection here. They're looking for patterns — consistent, ongoing need. If you need help often enough that it affects your independence, A&A may apply.

Housebound Benefits

Housebound benefits are for Veterans who can't leave their home very often due to a permanent disability. This doesn't mean you're literally trapped inside or that stepping onto the porch disqualifies you. It simply means your disability limits your ability to travel beyond your home or immediate surroundings.

A Veteran may qualify for Housebound benefits if they:

- Have a permanent disability that substantially confines them to their home
- Rarely leave except for medical appointments or essential activities

Housebound is less about needing personal assistance and more about limited mobility or medical restrictions that keep you homebound most of the time.

A&A vs. Housebound: *What is the Difference?*

A&A is about needing help. Housebound is about being limited.

Both increase your monthly Pension amount, but you can only receive one at a time – whichever provides the higher benefit. The VA doesn't stack them like pancakes, even though many Veterans wish they did.

When and How These Apply

These benefits apply when your health or living situation changes in a way that increases your need for support. Many Veterans qualify for Pension long before they qualify for A&A or Housebound. Others qualify for both at the same time. There's no "*right*" order — it depends entirely on your circumstances.

To apply, you typically submit medical evidence showing your level of need. This can include:

- Doctor statements
- Caregiver notes
- Nursing home records
- Descriptions of daily limitations

The VA reviews the evidence and determines whether A&A or Housebound applies. If approved, your monthly Pension amount increases accordingly.

Why This Matters

For many Veterans and their families, A&A or Housebound benefits can be life-changing. They can help pay for in-home care, assisted living, or the extra support needed to stay safe and independent. These benefits exist because the VA recognizes that aging, disability, and long-term health needs can create financial strain — and they want to help ease that burden.

Now that we've covered the core Pension program and the additional support available through Aid & Attendance and Housebound benefits, it's worth stepping back to look at how Pension fits into the bigger picture of VA benefits. Many Veterans qualify for both Pension and Compensation, but the two programs serve very different purposes — and choosing the right one can make a significant difference.

Pension vs. Compensation: Choosing the Right Path

By now, you've seen that VA Pension and VA Compensation may look similar from a distance — both are monthly, tax-free payments from the VA — but up close, they're built for completely different purposes. This is where many Veterans get tripped up. They hear "*VA benefit*," and assume everything works the same way. But choosing between Pension and Compensation is a bit like choosing between two roads that lead in different directions. The right one depends entirely on your circumstances.

The simplest way to understand the difference is this:

- Compensation is about what happened to you because of your service.
- Pension is about your financial situation after your service.

Compensation asks whether your disability is connected to your time in uniform. Pension asks whether you served during a wartime period and now have limited income or resources. One is tied to service-connected conditions; the other is tied to financial need.

Because the two programs serve different missions, you can technically qualify for both — but you can only receive **one** at a time. The VA will pay whichever benefit is higher, and in most cases, Compensation pays more. But that doesn't mean Pension is less important. For many wartime Veterans who don't have service-connected disabilities, Pension can be a lifeline.

Here's a simple way to think about the decision:

- If your disabilities were caused or worsened by your military service, Compensation is usually the right path.
- If your income is limited, you served during a wartime period, and you meet the age or disability requirements, Pension may be the better fit.
- If you qualify for both, the VA will automatically award the higher benefit — but understanding the differences helps you know what to expect.

Some Veterans start with Compensation and later transition to Pension as their financial or health situation changes. Others begin with Pension and later discover they qualify for Compensation after gathering more evidence or receiving new diagnoses. There's no "*wrong*" order. What matters is choosing the benefit that best supports your needs at the time.

The key takeaway is this: Compensation and Pension are not competing programs — they're complementary tools. One recognizes the cost of your service. The other provides a safety net when life becomes financially difficult. Knowing which one applies to you is the first step toward getting the support you've earned.

Understanding the difference between Compensation and Pension is a major milestone, and by now you've built a solid foundation for navigating the VA's financial support programs. But knowing what these benefits are is only half the journey. The next step — and the one that often feels the most intimidating — is preparing to actually file a claim.

This is where many Veterans start to feel overwhelmed. They wonder what evidence they need, whether their records are enough, how to explain their conditions, or whether they're missing something important. The good news is that filing a strong claim isn't about being perfect — it's about being prepared.

In the next chapter, we'll walk through the building blocks of a successful claim: gathering the right evidence, understanding the importance of a Nexus, using Disability Benefits Questionnaires effectively, and avoiding the common pitfalls that slow Veterans down. Think of this chapter as your pre-mission checklist — the part that ensures you're ready before you ever step onto the field.

† † † † †

If you're helping a Veteran with daily activities,
your time may count as a deductible medical expense —
even if you're a family member.

† † † † †

§ § § EXTRA INSIGHTS § § §

The VA Pension program can feel distant or irrelevant—right up until the moment it becomes essential. Here's something many Veterans never realize: Pension eligibility isn't fixed. It shifts as life shifts. A change in medical expenses, care needs, or household income can suddenly open a door that was closed before. That's why it's worth revisiting Pension from time to time, even if you once assumed you wouldn't qualify.

INSIDER TIP: *When the VA calculates Pension, they don't just look at income—they look at countable income. Many medical and care-related costs can reduce that number dramatically. Veterans and families often discover they qualify only after someone takes a second look with the right information. Keeping Pension on your radar ensures you won't miss support you've earned when you need it most.*

§ § § § § § § § §

Preparing to File

COMMON PITFALL:

Waiting until everything is "perfect" before filing.
Perfect is the enemy of progress —
and it can cost you months of benefits.

Before you ever fill out a form there's important groundwork to lay. Preparing to file isn't busywork—it's how you turn a confusing process into a clear, manageable plan. This chapter walks you through what to gather, what to think about, and how to organize your information so that when you do file, you're not guessing—you're ready.

Gathering Evidence

Before you ever click "*submit*" on a VA claim, there's one thing that will make or break your success more than anything else: evidence. The VA doesn't make decisions based on gut feelings, assumptions, or how convincing your story sounds. They make decisions based on what's in the record. That means the stronger your evidence, the stronger your claim.

Gathering evidence isn't about drowning the VA in paperwork. It's about collecting the right pieces — the ones that clearly show what happened, how it affects you today, and why it's connected to your service. Think of it like assembling a puzzle. Each piece matters, but only when they fit together do you get the full picture.

Most claims rely on three main types of evidence: service records, medical records, and buddy statements.

Service Records

Your service records help establish the "*when*" and "*where*" of your claim. They show your duty assignments, deployments, training, injuries, exposures, and anything else that ties your condition to your time in uniform. These records don't need to tell your entire life story — they just need to support the connection between your service and your condition.

For example, if you're filing for a knee injury, your service records might show a documented injury, physical training incidents, or duty assignments that involved repetitive stress. If you're filing for hearing loss, your records might show exposure to aircraft, artillery, or other high-noise environments.

Medical Records

Medical records are the backbone of your claim. They show the diagnosis, the severity of your condition, and how it affects your daily life. These can come from:

- VA medical centers
- Private doctors
- Specialists
- Urgent care or emergency visits

You don't need to be a medical expert — you just need to gather the records that show what's going on with your health. The VA will review them, compare them to the rating criteria, and determine how your condition fits into the VASRD.

Buddy Statements

Buddy statements are one of the most underrated tools in the entire VA system. These are written statements from people who served with you, lived with you, or witnessed your condition firsthand. They can fill in gaps when service records are incomplete or when an event wasn't formally documented.

A good buddy statement can:

- Confirm an injury or incident
- Describe changes in your behavior or health
- Support your account of what happened

They don't need to be fancy. They just need to be honest, specific, and signed.

Putting It All Together

When you gather service records, medical records, and buddy statements, you're building a clear, consistent story. You're showing the VA:

- What happened
- How it affects you now
- Why it's connected to your service

That's the heart of a strong claim. And once you have these pieces in place, you're ready for the next step — understanding the importance of a Nexus, which we'll explore in the next section.

Gathering evidence is the foundation of a strong claim, but evidence alone isn't enough. The VA also needs to understand *why* your current condition is connected to your military service. That connection — the bridge between "*what happened then*" and "*what's happening now*" — is called a Nexus. It's one of the most important parts of any claim, and it's where many Veterans either shine or stumble. In the next section, we'll break down what a Nexus is, why it matters, and how to make sure yours is as strong as possible.

---

† † † † †

The VA doesn't expect you to remember
exact dates from 15 years ago.
"Around 2008" or "during my second deployment"
is perfectly acceptable.

† † † † †

The Importance of a Nexus

If evidence is the backbone of your claim, the Nexus is the heartbeat. It's the part that brings everything to life — the explanation that ties your current disability to your time in service. Without a Nexus, the VA sees two separate events: something that happened in the past, and something you're dealing with now. The Nexus is what connects the dots.

A Nexus is simply a medical opinion stating that your current condition is "*at least as likely as not*" related to your military service. That phrase — *at least as likely as not* — is the VA's magic language. It means a 50/50 chance. It doesn't require certainty. It doesn't require absolute proof. It just requires a medically supported opinion that your condition is reasonably connected to your service.

Why the Nexus Matters

You can have perfect service records and detailed medical records, but without a Nexus, the VA may still deny your claim. That's because the VA needs a medical professional to explain the relationship between the two. The Nexus answers the question:

"Is your current disability connected to your military service?"

If the answer is yes — and it's supported by evidence — your claim becomes significantly stronger.

Strong vs. Weak Nexus Statements

Not all Nexus statements are created equally. Some are clear, detailed, and persuasive. Others are vague, incomplete, or unhelpful. Here's the difference:

A Strong Nexus Statement:

- Uses the VA's required language ("*at least as likely as not*")
- Explains why the condition is connected to service
- References medical records, service records, or known exposures
- Shows medical reasoning, not just a conclusion

Example of a Strong Nexus:

"*Based on the Veteran's documented knee injury during active duty in 2004, the chronic pain and reduced mobility noted in current examinations, and the absence of any significant post-service injuries, it is at least as likely as not that the Veteran's current left knee condition is related to military service.*"

This tells the VA what happened, why it matters, and how the doctor reached the conclusion.

A Weak Nexus Statement:

- Avoids the required language
- Offers no explanation
- Uses phrases like "*could be related*" or "*possibly connected*"
- Doesn't reference evidence

Example of a Weak Nexus:

"*The Veteran's knee pain may be related to service.*"

This is the medical equivalent of shrugging. The VA can't use it.

Who Can Provide a Nexus?

A Nexus must come from a medical professional. This can include:

- VA doctors
- Private physicians
- Specialists
- Nurse practitioners or physician assistants (*depending on state rules*)

You don't need a celebrity doctor or a 20-page report. You just need a clear, medically supported opinion.

When a Nexus Isn't Needed

Some conditions don't require a Nexus because the VA presumes they're related to service. These are called presumptive conditions, and we'll cover them in more detail later. For now, just know that if your condition falls under a presumptive category, the VA skips the Nexus step entirely.

Putting It All Together

A strong Nexus ties your evidence together and gives the VA a clear, medically supported reason to approve your claim. It's one of the most powerful tools you have — and understanding how it works puts you miles ahead of where most Veterans start.

In the next section, we'll look at another tool that can strengthen your claim even further: Disability Benefits Questionnaires (DBQs) — what they are, who completes them, and how they can help you present your condition clearly and confidently.

Disability Benefits Questionnaires (DBQs)

If the Nexus is the bridge between your service and your condition, the DBQ is the map that shows the VA exactly where you are today. A Disability Benefits Questionnaire is a standardized form the VA uses to evaluate the severity of your disability. Think of it as a checklist that helps medical providers describe your symptoms in the exact language the VA needs to rate your condition accurately.

DBQs don't replace medical records or Nexus opinions — they complement them. They take all the medical details that might be scattered across years of appointments and put them into one clear, organized document the VA can easily review.

What DBQs Are Designed to Do

A DBQ helps the VA understand:

- Your diagnosis
- Your symptoms
- How your condition affects your daily life
- How severe your limitations are
- Whether your condition has worsened over time

Each DBQ is tailored to a specific condition — there are DBQs for back problems, migraines, PTSD, hearing loss, knee injuries, respiratory issues, and dozens more. The VA uses these forms because they align directly with the rating criteria in the VASRD. In other words, DBQs speak the VA's language.

Who Completes a DBQ

A DBQ must be completed by a qualified medical professional. This can include:

- VA doctors
- Private physicians
- Specialists
- Nurse practitioners or physician assistants (*depending on state rules*)

You don't have to rely solely on VA providers. In fact, many Veterans choose to have a private doctor complete their DBQ because private providers often have more time to give a thorough, detailed evaluation.

How DBQs Strengthen Your Claim

A well-completed DBQ can:

- Provide clear evidence of the severity of your condition
- Reduce the need for additional VA exams
- Speed up the decision process
- Ensure the VA doesn't overlook key symptoms
- Support increases for worsening conditions

Because DBQs follow the VA's rating structure, they help prevent misunderstandings or missing information. They also give you a chance to present your condition in a structured, organized way – something that can make a real difference in how your claim is evaluated.

What Makes a Strong DBQ

A strong DBQ is:

- Complete — no skipped sections
- Specific — detailed descriptions, not vague statements
- Consistent — matches your medical records and symptoms
- Accurate — reflects your true limitations, not just your *"good days"*

A weak DBQ, on the other hand, may leave out important details, skip key questions, or fail to describe how your condition affects your daily life. The VA can only rate what's written down, so completeness matters.

DBQs and C&P Exams

Even with a DBQ, the VA may still schedule a Compensation and Pension (C&P) exam. This isn't a sign that anything is wrong — it's simply the VA's way of confirming the information. A strong DBQ can make that exam smoother and more accurate because the examiner already has a clear picture of your condition.

Putting It All Together

DBQs are one of the most effective tools you can use to strengthen your claim. They help the VA understand your condition in a structured, standardized way and ensure your symptoms are evaluated according to the correct criteria. When combined with solid evidence and a strong Nexus, a DBQ can significantly improve your chances of receiving the rating you deserve.

In the next section, we'll look at the common pitfalls Veterans run into during the claims process — and how to avoid them so your claim stays on track.

Common Pitfalls to Avoid

Even the most prepared Veteran can run into trouble during the claims process. The VA system has a lot of moving parts, and small oversights can create big delays. The good news is that most of these pitfalls are completely avoidable once you know what to look for. Think of this section as your "*heads-up display*" — the warnings that help you stay on course.

Missing or Incomplete Documents

One of the most common reasons claims get delayed is missing paperwork. The VA can't make a decision without the right records, and they won't guess or assume anything that isn't clearly documented.

Common missing items include:

- Service treatment records
- Private medical records
- Nexus letters
- DBQs
- Supporting evidence for secondary conditions

If the VA has to go hunting for documents, your claim slows down. If they can't find them at all, your claim may be denied. The solution is simple: gather everything up front and double-check that it's complete.

Vague or Unclear Claims

Another common pitfall is filing a claim that's too vague. Statements like "*back problems*," "*mental health issues*," or "*joint pain*" don't give the VA enough information to work with. The VA needs to know:

- What condition are you claiming
- When it began
- How it connects to your service
- How it affects you today

You don't need to write a novel – just be clear and specific. A well-defined claim is easier for the VA to evaluate and harder for them to misunderstand.

Not Describing How the Condition Affects Daily Life

Many Veterans focus on the diagnosis but forget to explain the impact. The VA rates disabilities based on functional loss – how your condition affects your ability to work, move, think, or perform daily activities.

If you don't describe:

- Pain levels
- Limitations
- Frequency of symptoms
- Impact on work or daily tasks

...the VA may underestimate the severity of your condition. This is where DBQs, medical records, and personal statements all work together.

Missing Deadlines

The VA has deadlines for appeals, supplemental claims, and certain types of evidence submissions. Missing a deadline doesn't always end your claim, but it can reset the process or force you to start over.

A few key deadlines include:

- One year to appeal a decision
- 90 days to submit evidence after certain requests
- Timelines for Higher-Level Reviews and Board appeals

Staying organized – even with a simple folder or checklist – can save you months of frustration.

Assuming the VA Will "*Fill in the Gaps*"

This is a big one. Many Veterans assume the VA will:

- Request every record (*even though the VA will request records they know about, not all providers respond or send complete files)*
- Interpret symptoms correctly
- Understand the connection between conditions
- Automatically consider secondary issues

The VA does have a legal duty to assist, which includes requesting medical and service records you identify, reviewing the evidence you submit, and developing your claim based on what's in the file. But that duty has limits. The VA can only work with the information they actually receive, and private providers don't always respond to VA requests—or send complete records.

Likewise, examiners and raters won't infer symptom severity, assume connections between conditions, or automatically consider secondary issues unless those things are clearly documented. This is why it's still the Veteran's responsibility to make sure the VA has the full picture: the right records, clear explanations of symptoms, and evidence showing how conditions relate. If something isn't documented, explained, or supported, the VA won't fill in the blanks for you.

Not Preparing for the C&P Exam

Even with strong evidence, the Compensation & Pension exam can make or break a claim. Many Veterans downplay symptoms, try to "*tough it out,*" or assume the examiner already knows their history.

A few reminders:

- Be honest
- Be specific
- Don't minimize your symptoms
- Describe your worst days, not your best ones

The C&P exam is a snapshot — make sure it reflects your real experience.

Putting It All Together

Avoiding these pitfalls doesn't require perfection — just awareness. When you gather complete evidence, write clear claims, stay organized, and prepare for the C&P exam, you dramatically increase your chances of a smooth, successful process.

Now that you know what to avoid, you're ready for the next major step: actually filing your claim. In the next chapter, we'll walk through the filing process step-by-step so you can move forward with confidence.

Filing Your Claim

Many Veterans file too narrowly. If a condition affects multiple parts of your life or causes new issues, include those in your claim.

This is where preparation turns into action. Filing your claim is more than just entering information into a form; it's how you present your story to the VA. In this chapter, we'll walk step-by-step through the filing process, explain key choices you'll make along the way, and show you how to file in a way that gives the VA what it needs to make a fair decision.

Step-by-Step Filing Process

Filing a VA claim isn't about being perfect — it's about being clear, organized, and intentional. Once you've prepared your evidence, the actual filing process becomes much easier. The VA gives you several ways to submit a claim, and each one has its own strengths. The key is choosing the method that works best for you and making sure your submission tells a complete, consistent story.

Here's a straightforward walkthrough of the filing process, from start to finish.

Step 1:
Choose How You Want to File

You have three main options:

- VA.gov — The most common and user-friendly method.
- Paper forms — Still valid, especially for Veterans who prefer physical documents.
- Accredited representatives — VSOs, accredited agents, or attorneys who can file on your behalf.

There's no "*best*" option — just the one that fits your comfort level. VA.gov is fast and convenient, but some Veterans prefer the reassurance of working with a trained representative.

Step 2:
Start Your Intent to File (Optional but Helpful)

If you're not ready to submit your full claim yet, you can start an Intent to File. This locks in your effective date – meaning the VA will pay back to that date once your claim is approved. It gives you time to gather evidence without losing potential benefits.

You can start an Intent to File through:

- VA.gov
- Calling the VA
- Submitting the appropriate form

It's quick, simple, and protects your timeline.

Step 3:
Complete the Application

For most disability claims, you'll use VA Form 21-526EZ. Whether you're filing online or on paper, the form will ask for:

- Your personal information
- Your service history
- The conditions you're claiming
- Supporting evidence
- Information about dependents (*if applicable*)

Be clear and specific when listing your conditions. Avoid vague terms like "*back issues*" or "*mental health problems.*" The VA needs to know exactly what you're claiming.

Step 4:
Upload or Submit Your Evidence

This is where all your preparation pays off. Upload:

- Service records
- Medical records
- Nexus letters
- DBQs
- Buddy statements
- Any other supporting documents

If you're filing through VA.gov, you can upload everything directly. If you're filing on paper, include copies — never originals.

Step 5:
Review and Submit

Before you hit "*submit,*" take a moment to review your claim:

- Are all documents attached?
- Are your conditions clearly listed?
- Does your evidence tell a consistent story?
- Are your Nexus statements strong and complete?

Once everything looks good, submit your claim. You'll receive a confirmation number or receipt, depending on the method you used.

Step 6:
Wait for the VA to Begin Review

After submission, the VA will:

- Acknowledge your claim
- Request any missing records
- Schedule a C&P exam (*if needed*)
- Begin reviewing your evidence

This part takes time but staying organized and responsive will help keep things moving.

But what if you file your claim and then realize you forgot to include a condition? You can add new conditions after submitting your claim, even if the VA hasn't issued a decision yet. Just be aware that adding conditions mid-process can slow things down. Each new issue requires its own development—records requests, exams, and review—which can extend the overall timeline. It's often better to submit everything together at the start, but if you discover something important later, it's still worth adding. The key is understanding that doing so may reset the clock or add extra steps before the VA can finish your claim(s).

Putting It All Together

Filing your claim is the moment where preparation meets action. When you've gathered strong evidence, built a clear Nexus, and organized your documents, the filing process becomes far less stressful. You're not just sending paperwork into the void — you're presenting a well-supported case that gives the VA everything they need to make a fair decision.

In the next section, we'll look at practical tips to help your claim stand out for all the right reasons and avoid the common mistakes that slow Veterans down.

---

† † † † †

You can upload evidence after you file.
Don't wait to submit your claim just because
you're still gathering documents.

† † † † †

Tips for Success

Filing a VA claim is part preparation, part communication, and part strategy. You don't need to be a legal expert or a medical professional — you just need to understand how to present your information in a way that helps the VA make a fair and accurate decision. These tips are designed to give you an edge, reduce frustration, and keep your claim moving smoothly.

Be Clear and Specific

The VA reviews thousands of claims every year. The clearer your claim is, the easier it is for them to understand what you're asking for. Avoid vague descriptions like "*back issues*" or "*mental health problems.*" Instead, be specific:

- "*Lumbar strain with chronic pain*"
- "*Generalized anxiety disorder with panic attacks*"
- "*Left knee instability following documented injury in service*"

Specificity helps the VA match your condition to the correct rating criteria.

Tell a Consistent Story

Your service records, medical records, Nexus letters, DBQs, and personal statements should all point in the same direction. They don't have to be identical, but they should support the same timeline and the same connection to service.

Inconsistencies — even small ones — can slow down your claim or raise questions the VA has to investigate.

Use Plain Language

You don't need to write like a lawyer. In fact, the VA often prefers simple, direct explanations. When describing your symptoms or limitations, focus on:

- What you experience
- How often it happens
- How it affects your daily life

Plain language is powerful because it's easy to understand and hard to misinterpret.

Document Functional Impact

The VA rates disabilities based on how they affect your ability to function, not just the diagnosis itself. When describing your condition, include details like:

- Difficulty standing, sitting, or walking
- Trouble concentrating or sleeping
- Pain levels and flare-ups
- Impact on work or daily tasks

This helps the VA understand the real-world impact of your condition.

Stay Organized

A simple folder — digital or physical — can save you hours of frustration. Keep copies of:

- All forms you submit
- All evidence you upload
- Notes from medical appointments
- Letters from the VA
- Deadlines and reminders

Staying organized helps you respond quickly if the VA requests additional information.

Respond Promptly to VA Requests

If the VA asks for more evidence or schedules a C&P exam, respond as soon as possible. Delays on your end can slow the entire process. Quick responses keep your claim moving.

Don't Minimize Your Symptoms

Many Veterans have a habit of "*toughing it out.*" But when you're filing a claim, honesty matters. Describe your symptoms as they truly are — not how you wish they were, and not how they are on your best days.

You're not complaining. You're documenting.

Consider Working with an Accredited Representative

VSOs, accredited agents, and attorneys can help you:

- Organize your evidence
- Submit your claim
- Understand VA language
- Avoid common mistakes

You don't have to do this alone. A good representative can make the process smoother and less stressful.

Putting It All Together

Success in the VA claims process isn't about luck — it's about clarity, consistency, and preparation. When you present your claim in a way that's easy for the VA to understand, you increase your chances of a faster, more accurate decision.

In the next section, we'll look at special considerations that apply to certain types of claims — including secondary conditions, presumptive conditions, and exposures like Agent Orange and Gulf War illnesses.

Special Considerations

Not all VA claims follow the same path. Some conditions are easier to prove because the VA already recognizes the connection to service. Others require a different type of evidence or a slightly different strategy. Knowing which category your condition falls into can make the entire process smoother and more predictable.

This section covers three major areas where Veterans often have questions: secondary conditions, presumptive conditions, and exposure-related conditions such as Gulf War illnesses and Agent Orange.

Secondary Conditions

A secondary condition is a disability that develops because of another service-connected condition. This is one of the most powerful — and most underused — parts of the VA system.

For example:

- A Veteran with a service-connected knee injury develops hip or back problems from years of altered movement.
- A Veteran with PTSD develops sleep apnea or migraines.
- A Veteran taking medication for a service-connected condition develops side effects like weight gain or gastrointestinal issues.

In each case, the secondary condition may also be eligible for service connection — not because it happened in service, but because it was caused or aggravated by a condition that *is* service-connected.

What You Need for a Secondary Claim

You'll need:

- Evidence of the primary service-connected condition
- A diagnosis of the secondary condition
- A Nexus showing the connection between the two

The Nexus is key. It must clearly state that the secondary condition is "*at least as likely as not*" caused or aggravated by the primary condition.

---

† † † † †

The VA can't rate what it doesn't know.
Be clear, be honest, and don't leave out details
because you think they're "not a big deal."

† † † † †

Presumptive Conditions

Presumptive conditions are the VA's way of saying, *"We already know this condition is connected to service under certain circumstances — you don't have to prove the Nexus."*

This can dramatically simplify and speed up your claim. Presumptive categories include:

- Agent Orange exposure
- Gulf War illnesses
- Burn pit exposure (*PACT Act*)
- Certain chronic conditions that appear within one year of discharge
- Radiation-exposed Veterans

If your condition falls under a presumptive category and you meet the service requirements, the VA automatically assumes the connection.

What You Need for a Presumptive Claim

You'll need:

- Proof of service in the qualifying location or era
- A diagnosis of the presumptive condition

You do <u>not</u> need a Nexus — the VA provides it for you.

Gulf War, Agent Orange, and Other Exposure-Related Claims

Some conditions are tied to specific exposures during service. These claims can be more complex, but they also come with special rules that can work in your favor.

Gulf War Illnesses

Gulf War Veterans may qualify for conditions that are:

- Chronic
- Medically unexplained
- Affecting multiple systems

These conditions don't require a traditional Nexus – the VA recognizes that many Gulf War illnesses don't have clear medical explanations.

Agent Orange

Veterans exposed to Agent Orange (*Vietnam, Korea DMZ, certain ships, and now expanded locations under the PACT Act*) qualify for a long list of presumptive conditions, including:

- Diabetes
- Ischemic heart disease
- Certain cancers
- Parkinson's disease

Again, no Nexus required—just proof of service in a qualifying area.

Burn Pits and Toxic Exposures (*PACT Act*)

The PACT Act expanded presumptive conditions for Veterans exposed to burn pits and other toxins. This includes many respiratory conditions and cancers.

If you served in a qualifying location during a qualifying period, the VA presumes exposure.

Putting It All Together

Special considerations can make your claim easier — but only if you know how they apply to your situation. Secondary conditions require a strong Nexus. Presumptive conditions skip the Nexus entirely. Exposure-related claims may fall into either category depending on your service.

Understanding these differences helps you file smarter, avoid unnecessary hurdles, and give the VA exactly what they need to approve your claim.

In the next section, we'll look at the important role family members can play in the claims process — from gathering evidence to offering support during exams and decisions.

---

† † † † †

When describing your condition,
focus on frequency, severity, and impact.
These three details help the
VA understand the real picture.

† † † † †

Family Member Roles

Filing a VA claim isn't just a paperwork exercise — it's a life event. It affects the Veteran, the household, and often the people who provide day-to-day support. Family members and caregivers can play a crucial role in helping the Veteran stay organized, gather evidence, and communicate clearly with the VA. Their involvement doesn't replace the Veteran's voice — it amplifies it.

Here are the most common and most helpful ways family members can support the process.

Helping Gather Evidence

Family members often have access to information the Veteran may overlook:

- Old medical records
- Deployment orders or service documents
- Photos, letters, or journals that show symptoms or injuries
- Notes from past appointments
- Medication lists

Sometimes the Veteran is too close to the situation to see what's important. A spouse or caregiver may remember details the Veteran forgot or didn't think mattered.

Providing Lay Statements

Family members can write lay statements — personal accounts describing what they've observed. These statements can be incredibly powerful, especially for conditions that affect behavior, mobility, sleep, mood, or daily functioning.

A strong family lay statement might describe:

- Changes in the Veteran's physical abilities
- Mood swings, anxiety, or depression
- Sleep disturbances
- Memory or concentration issues
- Pain levels and flare-ups
- How the condition affects work or home life

These statements help the VA understand the real-world impact of the disability — something medical records alone can't always capture.

Supporting the Veteran During C&P Exams

C&P exams can be stressful. Family members can help by:

- Driving the Veteran to the appointment
- Helping them remember key symptoms
- Encouraging them to be honest and specific
- Providing emotional support before and after

In some cases, examiners may allow a spouse or caregiver to attend part of the exam to offer context — especially for mental health or cognitive conditions.

Helping With Organization and Deadlines

The VA system involves:

- Forms
- Evidence uploads
- Letters
- Deadlines
- Requests for information

Family members can help keep everything organized, track dates, and ensure nothing slips through the cracks. A simple calendar or shared folder can make a big difference.

Communicating With Accredited Representatives

If the Veteran is working with a VSO, accredited agent, or attorney, family members can help:

- Ask questions
- Provide documents
- Clarify timelines
- Keep communication flowing

This is especially helpful when the Veteran is overwhelmed, dealing with health issues, or simply trying to keep track of everything.

Emotional Support

Filing a claim can bring up old memories, frustrations, or anxieties. Family members often play the most important role of all — offering patience, encouragement, and understanding. The process can be long, and having someone in your corner makes a world of difference.

Putting It All Together

Family members aren't just bystanders in the claims process — they're partners. Their support can strengthen the claim, reduce stress, and help the Veteran stay focused and organized. When everyone works together, the process becomes smoother, clearer, and far less overwhelming.

Now that you've prepared your claim and understand the filing process, it's time to look at what happens next. In the next chapter, we'll walk through the VA's review process, C&P exams, decision letters, and how to stay organized while you wait.

---

† † † † †

You can save your claim as a draft
and return to it anytime.
Filing doesn't have to be a one-sitting marathon.

† † † † †

§ § § EXTRA INSIGHTS § § §

Filing a VA claim can feel intimidating, but here's something most Veterans never hear: the strongest claims don't come from perfect paperwork—they come from Veterans who take a moment to get clear about their story. Before you submit anything, pause and write down the "big picture" of what you're claiming and why. That simple step does more than organize your thoughts; it helps the VA understand your experience without having to guess.

INSIDER TIP: *VA reviewers are trained to follow the evidence trail you give them. When your claim is clear, consistent, and supported—even with basic documentation—you make their job easier and your path smoother. A few minutes of preparation on your end can save weeks of back-and-forth later and often leads to a cleaner, faster decision.*

§ § § § § § § § §

After You File

The waiting period is where most Veterans start doubting themselves.
Don't!
You've done the hard part — now let the process work.

Once your claim is submitted, the waiting begins—and with it, a lot of questions. What is the VA doing? How long will it take? What should you be watching for? This chapter explains what happens behind the scenes after you file, how to track your claim, how to read VA letters, and what to do (*and not do*) while the decision is pending.

The VA Review Process

Once your claim is submitted, the VA begins a structured, multi-step review process. It may not always feel fast, but it *is* methodical – and understanding how it works can make the waiting period far less stressful. Think of this chapter as your behind-the-scenes tour of what the VA is doing while you're checking your mailbox or refreshing VA.gov.

The claim review process generally includes four major stages: initial review, evidence gathering, C&P exams, and decision preparation.

Initial Review

After your claim is received, the VA assigns it to a reviewer who performs a quick assessment. Their job is to:

- Confirm your claim is complete
- Identify what evidence is already included
- Determine what additional records may be needed
- Request service or medical records if they aren't already provided

This stage is usually fast – sometimes just a few days – but it sets the tone for everything that follows.

Evidence Gathering

Next, the VA begins collecting any missing information. This may include:

- Service treatment records
- VA medical records
- Private medical records (*if you authorized release*)
- Personnel records
- Exposure records (*Agent Orange, Gulf War, burn pits, etc.*)

If the VA needs something from you — additional evidence, clarification, or a form — they'll send a letter or update your VA.gov portal. Responding promptly helps keep your claim moving.

Compensation & Pension (C&P) Exams

Most claims require a C&P exam, which is the VA's opportunity to evaluate your condition directly. These exams are performed by VA clinicians or contracted providers.

During the exam, the examiner will:

- Review your medical history
- Ask questions about your symptoms
- Perform physical or psychological evaluations
- Complete a DBQ or similar assessment

The examiner does not make the final decision — they simply provide medical findings that the VA uses to rate your condition.

Review and Decision Preparation

Once all evidence is gathered and exams are complete, the VA:

- Reviews your entire file
- Applies the rating criteria
- Drafts a decision
- Prepares your notification letter

This stage can take time, especially if your claim involves multiple conditions or complex medical issues. But this is where everything comes together — your evidence, your Nexus, your DBQs, and your exam results.

Putting It All Together

The VA review process may feel slow, but it follows a clear structure. Understanding each step helps you stay grounded and reduces the anxiety that comes from not knowing what's happening behind the scenes.

In the next section, we'll break down the different types of VA decisions — approvals, partial approvals, and denials — and what each one means for your next steps.

---

† † † † †

You can upload additional evidence at any point
while your claim is open —
even if the VA hasn't asked for it yet.

† † † † †

Understanding VA Decisions

When the VA finishes reviewing your claim, they'll send you a decision letter explaining what they decided, why they decided it, and what happens next. These letters can look intimidating — lots of pages, legal language, and medical terminology — but once you understand the structure, they become much easier to navigate.

VA decisions generally fall into three categories: approval, partial approval, and denial.

Approval

An approval means the VA agrees that your condition is service-connected and has assigned a disability rating. Your decision letter will include:

- The conditions that were approved
- The percentage assigned to each condition
- The effective date
- Your monthly payment amount
- Whether future exams or re-evaluations are scheduled

Even with an approval, it's important to review the details carefully. Make sure:

- The effective date matches when you filed or when the condition worsened
- The rating accurately reflects the severity of your symptoms
- All conditions you claimed were addressed

If something seems incorrect, you still have options — which we'll cover in the appeals section.

Partial Approval

A partial approval means the VA approved some parts of your claim but not others. This is extremely common and can happen for several reasons:

- One condition is approved, another is denied
- A condition is approved but rated lower than expected
- A condition is approved but the effective date is later than you believe it should be

Partial approvals don't mean your claim was weak — they simply reflect how the VA interpreted the evidence for each condition. You can accept the approved portions while still appealing the parts you disagree with.

Denial

A denial means the VA did not find enough evidence to grant service connection or did not agree that your condition is related to your service. A denial can happen for reasons such as:

- No diagnosis
- No documented in-service event or injury
- No Nexus connecting the condition to service
- Insufficient evidence of severity
- Missing or incomplete records

A denial is not the end of the road. It simply means the VA needs more information or clearer evidence. Many Veterans successfully win their claims on appeal once they understand what the VA found lacking.

Understanding the "*Reasons for Decision*" Section

Every decision letter includes a section called Reasons for Decision. This is the VA's explanation of:

- What evidence they reviewed
- What they found persuasive
- What they found lacking
- Why they assigned the rating they did
- Why they denied or partially denied certain conditions

This section is incredibly important. It tells you exactly what the VA needs to approve your claim — and it guides your next steps if you choose to appeal.

Effective Dates

The effective date determines when your payments begin. It's usually:

- The date you filed your claim, or
- The date the VA received your Intent to File

If the effective date seems wrong, you may be entitled to back pay — and you can appeal that specific issue without reopening the entire claim.

What Happens Next

After receiving your decision letter, you have options:

- Accept the decision
- File a Supplemental Claim with new evidence
- Request a Higher-Level Review
- Appeal directly to the Board of Veterans' Appeals

You have **one year** from the date of the decision to choose your path. We'll explore these options in detail in the next section.

Putting It All Together

VA decisions can feel overwhelming, but they follow a clear structure. Whether your claim is approved, partially approved, or denied, the decision letter gives you valuable information about what the VA needs and what your next steps should be. Understanding the decision is the key to moving forward with confidence — whether that means accepting the outcome or preparing an appeal.

In the next section, we'll walk through the appeals process, including Higher-Level Reviews, Supplemental Claims, and Board appeals, so you know exactly how to respond if you disagree with the VA's decision.

Appeals & Higher-Level Reviews

If you disagree with the VA's decision, you're not alone – and you're not stuck. The modern VA appeals system, known as the AMA (*Appeals Modernization Act*), gives you three clear options to keep your claim moving forward. Each option serves a different purpose, and choosing the right one can make a major difference in the outcome.

Here are the three main appeal lanes:

- Higher-Level Review (HLR)
- Supplemental Claim
- Board of Veterans' Appeals (BVA)

Let's break them down in a way that makes sense.

Higher-Level Review (HLR)

A Higher-Level Review is exactly what it sounds like: a more experienced VA reviewer takes a fresh look at your claim. This is not a new claim – it's a second opinion based on the same evidence you have already submitted.

When to Choose HLR

HLR is a good option when:

- You believe the VA made a mistake
- The evidence was strong, but the decision didn't reflect it
- The VA misinterpreted or overlooked something

HLR is <u>not</u> the right choice if you have new evidence – the VA will not consider anything new in this lane.

What Makes HLR Unique

- You can request an informal conference — a phone call where you or your representative can point out errors or clarify issues.
- A more senior reviewer handles your case.
- The decision is usually faster than other appeal options.

HLR is about correcting errors, <u>not</u> adding evidence.

Supplemental Claim

A Supplemental Claim is the right choice when you have new and relevant evidence that wasn't part of your original claim.

Examples of New and Relevant Evidence

- A new medical opinion or Nexus letter
- Updated DBQs
- Private medical records the VA didn't have
- Buddy statements
- Evidence the VA failed to obtain the first time

"*New and relevant*" doesn't mean "*perfect*." It just needs to add something meaningful to your case.

When to Choose a Supplemental Claim

Choose this lane when:

- You were denied due to lack of evidence
- Your rating was too low
- You've gathered stronger (*or additional*) medical support
- You want to build a more complete case

This is the most flexible appeal option and often the most successful when used correctly.

Board of Veterans' Appeals (BVA)

If you want a Veterans Law Judge to review your case, the Board appeal is your path. This is the most formal option – and often the slowest – but it can be the most powerful when your case needs deeper review.

Three Board Options

Direct Review

- No new evidence
- No hearing
- Judge reviews the existing record
- Fastest Board option

Evidence Submission

- You can submit new evidence within 90 days
- No hearing

Hearing Lane

- You meet with a Veterans Law Judge (*virtual or in-person*)
- You can submit new evidence
- Longest timeline, but sometimes necessary

When to Choose a Board Appeal

- The VA misapplied the law
- Your case is complex
- You want a judge to weigh the evidence
- You need to present testimony
- Other lanes didn't resolve the issue

Board appeals take time, but they can be incredibly effective.

Timelines and Deadlines

You have one year from the date of your decision letter to choose any of the three appeal lanes. You can also switch lanes if needed — for example, filing a Supplemental Claim after an HLR.

The key is choosing the lane that matches your situation, not rushing into the first option you see.

Putting It All Together

Appeals aren't about starting over — they're about strengthening your case. Whether you need a second look, new evidence, or a judge's review, the VA gives you multiple paths to keep moving forward. Understanding these options helps you make informed decisions and stay in control of your claim.

In the next section, we'll look at how to stay organized and steady during the waiting period — a stage that can test your patience but doesn't have to derail your progress.

---

† † † † †

The VA can't move forward without your response.
If they ask for something, reply as soon as you can.

† † † † †

Staying Organized During the Wait

Once your claim or appeal is in motion, the waiting begins – and this is where many Veterans feel the most frustration. You've done your part, submitted your evidence, and followed the steps. Now the process shifts to the VA's timeline, which can feel slow or unpredictable. Staying organized during this period helps you stay in control, reduces stress, and ensures you're ready for whatever comes next.

Here are the most effective ways to stay organized and steady while you wait.

Keep All Your Documents in One Place

Whether you prefer digital folders, a binder, or a simple envelope, having everything together makes a huge difference. Keep copies of:

- Your claim or appeal forms
- All evidence you submitted
- C&P exam notes (*your own notes or summaries*)
- VA letters and notifications
- Deadlines and reminders

This becomes your "*VA command center*" – a single place where nothing gets lost.

Track Deadlines and Requests

The VA may send:

- Requests for more evidence
- Notices of scheduled exams
- Updates on your claim status
- Letters explaining next steps

Missing a deadline can slow your claim or force you to restart a process. A simple calendar — digital or paper — can keep everything on track.

Check VA.gov Periodically (*But Not Constantly*)

VA.gov is the most reliable way to track your claim's progress. Checking it once a week is usually enough. Checking it every day can drive you crazy — the status doesn't change that fast.

Look for updates like:

- "*Evidence gathering*"
- "*Review of evidence*"
- "*Preparation for decision*"
- "*Pending decision approval*"

These stages help you understand where your claim is in the process.

Keep Notes After Every Appointment

If you have medical appointments, therapy sessions, or new symptoms, jot down a few notes. These can help:

- Support future claims or increases
- Strengthen appeals
- Refresh your memory during exams
- Provide clarity to your representative

You don't need a diary — just a few lines about what happened and how you felt.

Stay in Touch with Your Representative

VSOs, accredited agents, and attorneys can:

- Check the status of your claim
- Interpret VA letters
- Help you respond to requests
- Prepare you for exams or appeals

A quick check-in every few weeks keeps communication flowing and prevents surprises.

Prepare for Possible Next Steps

While you wait, it helps to think ahead:

- If you're expecting a C&P exam, review your symptoms and limitations.
- If you're expecting a decision, review your evidence so you're ready to interpret the results.
- If you're considering an appeal, start gathering any additional evidence you might need.

Preparation reduces stress and keeps you proactive, not reactive.

Take Care of Yourself

This process can be emotionally draining. It's okay to feel frustrated or anxious — many Veterans do. Staying organized helps, but so does:

- Talking with family or friends
- Taking breaks from thinking about the claim
- Focusing on hobbies or routines
- Remembering that waiting is part of the process, not a sign of failure

You're doing the right thing by pursuing the benefits you've earned.

Putting It All Together

Staying organized during the waiting period doesn't just help you keep track of paperwork — it helps you stay grounded. When you know where everything is, what's coming next, and how to respond to the VA, the entire process becomes more manageable. You can't control the VA's timeline, but you *can* control how prepared you are.

Now that you understand what happens after you file — and how to stay steady during the wait — it's time to shift gears. In the next chapter, we'll explore how to maximize your benefits, including secondary service connections, Special Monthly Compensation, survivor benefits, and how VA benefits interact with other programs.

Maximizing Your Benefits

Some of the biggest rating increases come from conditions Veterans didn't even realize were connected — migraines from neck injuries, depression from chronic pain, sleep apnea linked to PTSD, and more.

Getting a decision is not always the end of the story. Sometimes there are additional benefits you qualify for, conditions that should be rated higher, or secondary issues that haven't been claimed yet. This chapter focuses on making sure you're not leaving anything on the table—exploring increases, secondary claims, special monthly compensation, and other ways to ensure your benefits truly reflect your situation.

Secondary Service Connections

A secondary service connection is one of the most powerful — and most overlooked — tools in the entire VA system. Many Veterans focus only on the conditions that began in service, but the VA also recognizes that disabilities don't exist in isolation. One condition can cause or worsen another, and when that happens, the second condition may also be eligible for service connection.

Think of your primary service-connected condition as the first domino. When it falls, it can set off a chain reaction — and the VA allows you to claim those downstream effects.

What Counts as a Secondary Condition?

A secondary condition is any disability that is:

- Caused by a service-connected condition, or
- Aggravated by a service-connected condition

This includes physical, mental, and even medication-related issues (*for treatment of service-connected conditions*).

Common Examples

- A Veteran with a service-connected knee injury develops hip or back problems from years of altered gait.
- A Veteran with PTSD develops sleep apnea, migraines, or gastrointestinal issues.
- A Veteran with diabetes develops neuropathy or kidney problems.
- A Veteran taking medication for chronic pain develops depression or weight-related conditions.

If the primary condition is service-connected, the secondary condition may be too — even if it didn't begin during service.

Why Secondary Claims Matter

Secondary conditions can:

- Increase your overall combined rating
- Provide access to additional benefits
- Recognize the full impact of your service-connected disabilities
- Strengthen future claims or appeals

Many Veterans qualify for higher ratings through secondary conditions than through their primary conditions alone.

---

† † † † †

SERVICE CONNECTION means the VA agrees your disability is linked to your military service. Without it, compensation can't begin — with it, everything becomes possible.

† † † † †

What You Need to Prove a Secondary Condition

A strong secondary claim includes three key pieces:

- A current diagnosis of the secondary condition
- Evidence of the primary service-connected condition
- A Nexus linking the two

The Nexus must state that the secondary condition is "*at least as likely as not*" caused or aggravated by the primary condition.

Example of a Strong Secondary Nexus

"*Based on the Veteran's service-connected left knee instability and documented gait abnormalities, it is at least as likely as not that the Veteran's chronic lower back pain has been aggravated beyond its natural progression.*"

This ties everything together clearly and medically.

Aggravation vs. Causation

The VA recognizes two types of secondary connections:

- Causation: The primary condition directly caused the secondary condition.
- Aggravation: The primary condition made the secondary condition worse.

Aggravation claims are especially powerful because the secondary condition doesn't have to be caused by service — it only needs to be worsened by a service-connected disability.

Evidence That Strengthens Secondary Claims

Strong secondary claims often include:

- DBQs for both conditions
- Medical opinions explaining the connection
- Treatment notes showing progression
- Imaging or test results
- Lay statements describing changes over time

The more clearly you show the relationship, the stronger your claim becomes.

Putting It All Together

Secondary service connections allow the VA to recognize the full picture of your health — not just the conditions that began in service, but the ones that developed because of them. When used effectively, secondary claims can significantly increase your rating, improve your access to care, and ensure you're fully supported.

In the next section, we'll explore Special Monthly Compensation (SMC) — an additional benefit for Veterans whose disabilities create unique challenges or require extra support.

---

† † † † †

Veterans often go from confused and frustrated
to confident and successful —
not because the system changed,
but because they understood it.

† † † † †

Special Monthly Compensation (SMC)

Special Monthly Compensation is one of the most valuable — and most overlooked — benefits the VA offers. Unlike standard disability ratings, which focus on percentages, SMC provides additional tax-free compensation for Veterans whose disabilities create specific, serious limitations or require special assistance.

Think of SMC as the VA's way of saying: *"Your situation requires more support than the standard rating system can provide."*

SMC is not a separate claim type — it's an entitlement. If you qualify, the VA is supposed to grant it automatically. But in practice, many Veterans never receive it simply because they don't know it exists or don't recognize when they qualify.

What Is SMC?

SMC is extra compensation for Veterans who:

- Need help with daily activities
- Have severe disabilities affecting mobility or independence
- Have loss or loss of use of certain organs or limbs
- Are housebound
- Require aid and attendance
- Have combinations of disabilities that create exceptional circumstances

SMC is paid in addition to your regular disability compensation.

Common Types of SMC

There are many SMC levels, but here are the ones Veterans encounter most often.

SMC-K:
Loss or Loss of Use

This is the simplest and most common SMC level. It applies when a Veteran has:

- Loss or loss of use of a hand or foot
- Loss of use of reproductive organs
- Loss of hearing in both ears
- Loss of sight in one eye
- Loss of breast tissue (*common after cancer treatment*)

SMC-K can be added on top of any rating, even 100%.

SMC-S:
Housebound

SMC-S applies when:

- You have one disability rated at 100%, and
- You have additional disabilities that combine to 60% or more, or
- You are substantially confined to your home due to service-connected disabilities

Many Veterans qualify for SMC-S without realizing it — especially those with a single 100% rating plus multiple secondary conditions.

SMC-L Through SMC-O:
Aid and Attendance & Severe Disabilities

- These higher levels apply when a Veteran:
- Needs help with daily activities (*bathing, dressing, feeding, toileting*)
- Is bedridden
- Has severe mobility limitations
- Has loss of use of multiple limbs
- Has blindness or near-blindness
- Requires regular supervision for safety

Aid and Attendance is one of the most powerful forms of SMC and can significantly increase monthly compensation.

How to Qualify for SMC

You can qualify for SMC through:

- Medical evidence showing loss of use, mobility limitations, or need for assistance
- DBQs that document functional limitations
- Lay statements from family or caregivers
- C&P exams that confirm severity
- Existing ratings that meet SMC criteria

You do not need to file a separate claim for SMC. If the evidence supports it, the VA is required to grant it. However, many Veterans still submit a request to ensure the VA reviews the issue.

Why SMC Matters

SMC can:

- Increase your monthly compensation
- Recognize the full impact of severe disabilities
- Provide support for caregivers
- Improve quality of life
- Ensure long-term stability for you and your family

For some Veterans, SMC increases their benefits more than any rating increase ever could.

Putting It All Together

Special Monthly Compensation is one of the most important tools for ensuring Veterans receive the full support they've earned. Whether it's loss of use, housebound status, or the need for daily assistance, SMC recognizes the real-world challenges that standard ratings can't fully capture.

In the next section, we'll explore survivor benefits — including Dependency and Indemnity Compensation (DIC) — so your family understands what support is available if the unthinkable happens.

Dependency & Indemnity Compensation (DIC) for Survivors

Survivor benefits are some of the most important — and most compassionate — programs the VA offers. They exist to ensure that when a Veteran passes away, their family isn't left without support. These benefits can provide monthly compensation, access to healthcare, education assistance, and even help with burial costs.

The cornerstone of VA survivor benefits is Dependency and Indemnity Compensation (DIC), but it's not the only program available. Understanding these benefits now helps your family avoid confusion later and ensures they receive everything they're entitled to.

Dependency and Indemnity Compensation (DIC)

DIC is a tax-free monthly benefit paid to eligible survivors of:

- Veterans who died from a service-connected condition
- Veterans who were rated totally disabled (*100% or TDIU*) for a qualifying period before death
- Service members who died on active duty, active duty for training, or inactive duty training

DIC is one of the most significant benefits the VA provides to surviving spouses and dependents.

Who Is Eligible for DIC?

Surviving Spouses

A surviving spouse may qualify if:

- The Veteran died from a service-connected condition, or
- The Veteran was rated totally disabled (*100% or TDIU*) for:
    - 10 years before death, or
    - 5 years from discharge to death, or
    - 1 year if the Veteran was a former POW

Spouses may also qualify if they:

- Lived with the Veteran continuously until death (*with some exceptions*)
- Remarried after age 57 (*and in some cases after age 55*)

Dependent Children

Children may qualify if they are:

- Under age 18, or
- Between 18–23 and attending school, or
- Permanently incapable of self-support due to disability

Dependent Parents

In some cases, parents with financial need may qualify for Parents' DIC.

How DIC Is Awarded

DIC is awarded when:

- The Veteran's death certificate lists a service-connected condition as a primary or contributing cause, or
- Medical evidence shows a service-connected condition materially contributed to death, or
- The Veteran met the "*10-year rule*," "*5-year rule*," or POW rule for total disability

Survivors do not need to prove negligence or fault — only that the death was connected to service or that the Veteran met the qualifying disability period.

---

† † † † †

Your rating should reflect your reality.
If your symptoms limit your daily life
more than your rating suggests,
it's time to revisit your benefits.

† † † † †

Additional Survivor Benefits

DIC is the foundation, but survivors may also qualify for:

CHAMPVA (Healthcare)

Healthcare coverage for surviving spouses and dependents if the Veteran was rated permanently and totally disabled.

Survivors' and Dependents' Educational Assistance (DEA)

Education benefits for spouses and children, including:

- College
- Technical training
- Apprenticeships
- Career programs

Burial Benefits

These may include:

- Burial allowances
- Headstones or markers
- Presidential Memorial Certificates
- Burial in a VA national cemetery

Accrued Benefits

Unpaid benefits the Veteran was entitled to before death.

Survivor Pension

For low-income surviving spouses and children of wartime Veterans.

Why Understanding Survivor Benefits Matters

Survivor benefits:

- Provide financial stability
- Protect families from unexpected hardship
- Ensure long-term healthcare access
- Support education and career goals
- Honor the Veteran's service and sacrifice

Many families don't realize they qualify — or they apply too late. Understanding these benefits now ensures your loved ones are prepared.

Putting It All Together

Survivor benefits are a vital part of the VA system, offering support and stability when families need it most. DIC, CHAMPVA, DEA, and burial benefits can make a profound difference in the lives of surviving spouses and children. By understanding these programs now, you give your family clarity and confidence for the future.

In the next section, we'll explore how VA benefits interact with other programs — including Social Security, Medicare, and state-level benefits — so you can see the full picture of support available to you and your family.

Combining VA Benefits with Other Programs

VA disability compensation is just one part of the broader network of benefits available to Veterans. Many Veterans also qualify for Social Security programs, Medicare, state-level benefits, and even private insurance or retirement systems. Knowing how these programs interact can help you avoid misunderstandings and ensure you're receiving everything you've earned.

The good news is that VA disability compensation is one of the most flexible benefits out there — it rarely reduces or interferes with other programs. But there *are* important rules and exceptions to understand.

VA Disability and Social Security Disability (SSDI)

VA disability compensation does not reduce Social Security Disability Insurance (SSDI). You can receive both at the same time with no offset.

Key Points

- SSDI is based on your work history, not your disability rating.
- A 100% VA rating can strengthen your SSDI claim, but it doesn't guarantee approval.
- SSDI decisions and VA decisions are independent — one does not control the other.

Many Veterans receive both benefits without issue.

VA Disability and Social Security Retirement

VA disability compensation does not affect Social Security retirement benefits. You can receive both in full.

Important Note

- Your VA rating does not change your Social Security retirement amount.
- Your Social Security retirement does not reduce your VA compensation.

These two programs operate completely separately.

VA Disability and Medicare

Medicare eligibility is based on age (65+) or SSDI approval — not your VA rating.

How They Work Together

- You can have both VA healthcare and Medicare.
- Many Veterans use Medicare for civilian providers and VA for specialty care.
- Medicare Part B premiums are not affected by VA benefits.

Having both systems gives you more flexibility in choosing providers.

VA Disability and Medicaid

Medicaid is income-based, so VA disability may affect eligibility depending on your state.

General Rules

- VA disability compensation is usually counted as income for Medicaid.
- Some states exclude part or all of VA benefits when determining eligibility.
- Medicaid can work alongside VA healthcare for long-term care needs.

If long-term care is a concern, it's worth checking your state's rules.

VA Disability and State Veteran Benefits

Every state offers its own set of Veteran benefits, which may include:

- Property tax exemptions
- Free or discounted vehicle registration
- State Park access
- Tuition assistance
- Hunting and fishing licenses
- State Veteran homes

Many of these benefits require a minimum VA disability rating (*often 50%, 70%, or 100%*).

Key Tip

Your VA rating unlocks state benefits — but you must apply separately through your state's Veteran affairs office.

VA Disability and Military Retirement Pay

If you receive military retirement pay, VA disability compensation can interact with it in two ways:

Concurrent Retirement and Disability Pay (CRDP)

Allows you to receive both full military retirement and VA disability if you are:

- Rated 50% or higher, or
- Receiving combat-related special compensation

Combat-Related Special Compensation (CRSC)

Tax-free compensation for combat-related disabilities. You must apply through your branch of service.

These programs ensure you don't lose retirement income because of your VA rating.

VA Disability and Private Insurance

VA disability compensation:

- Does not affect private health insurance
- Does not reduce life insurance payouts
- Does not interfere with employer-provided benefits

In fact, some private insurers offer additional coverage for service-connected disabilities.

Putting It All Together

VA disability compensation is one of the most flexible benefits available — it rarely reduces or interferes with other programs. Instead, it often works alongside Social Security, Medicare, state benefits, and military retirement to create a stronger, more stable support system for you and your family.

Understanding how these programs interact helps you make informed decisions, avoid surprises, and ensure you're receiving every benefit you've earned.

In the next section, we'll look at common myths and misunderstandings about VA benefits — the kind of misinformation that causes Veterans to miss out on support or make decisions based on fear instead of facts.

---

† † † † †

If a condition has gotten worse,
you don't need to wait for your next appointment
to request an increase.
The VA rates your current level of disability,
not last year's.

† † † † †

Common Myths and Misunderstandings

The VA system is full of rules, timelines, and terminology — and where there's complexity, there are myths. Some of these myths come from outdated policies. Others come from misunderstandings passed from one Veteran to another. And some come from fear: fear of losing benefits, fear of being denied, or fear of doing something "*wrong*."

This section clears the air. Here are the most common myths Veterans encounter — and the truth behind them.

Myth #1:
"If I file a claim, the VA will reduce my current rating."

Truth:
Filing a new claim does *not* automatically trigger a review of your existing ratings. The VA only re-evaluates a condition if:

- You specifically request an increase, or
- There is clear evidence your condition has improved significantly

Most Veterans file new claims or secondary claims without any impact on their existing ratings.

Myth #2:
"I need to be 100% disabled to qualify for benefits."

Truth:
Even a 0% rating can unlock benefits, including:

- Healthcare
- Presumptive protections
- Secondary service connections

Every percentage matters. You don't need to be 100% to receive meaningful support.

Myth #3:
"If I'm working, I can't get VA disability."

Truth:

VA disability compensation is not income-based. You can work full-time, part-time, or not at all — your rating is based on your symptoms, not your employment.

The only exception is TDIU, which has specific work-related rules. Standard disability ratings do not.

Myth #4:
"If I get SSDI or Social Security, the VA will reduce my benefits."

Truth:

VA disability compensation does not reduce Social Security benefits, and Social Security does not reduce VA compensation. They are completely separate systems. You can receive both in full.

Myth #5:
"The VA will automatically find all my records."

Truth:

The VA tries — but they don't always succeed. Missing records are one of the most common reasons for delays or denials.

Providing your own:

- Service records
- Private medical records
- Nexus letters
- DBQs

...dramatically strengthens your claim.

Myth #6:
"If my condition wasn't documented in service, I can't get service-connected."

Truth:

Many conditions qualify even without in-service documentation, including:

- PTSD
- Hearing loss
- Migraines
- Secondary conditions
- Gulf War illnesses
- Toxic exposure conditions

A strong Nexus can bridge the gap.

Myth #7:
"I can only file one condition at a time."

Truth:

You can file:

- Multiple conditions
- Secondary conditions
- Increases
- Supplemental claims

...all at once. The VA will process them together.

Myth #8:
"If I miss a C&P exam, my claim is automatically denied."

Truth:

Missing an exam can delay your claim, but it's not an automatic denial. If you miss an exam:

- Call the VA immediately
- Explain the situation
- Request a reschedule

Most examiners will accommodate reasonable circumstances.

Myth #9:
"If I get DIC or survivor benefits, I lose Social Security or other support."

Truth:

DIC does not reduce Social Security, retirement, or most state benefits. It is tax-free and stands on its own.

Myth #10:
"The VA is out to deny my claim."

Truth:

The VA's job is to apply the law to the evidence. When claims are denied, it's usually because:

- Evidence is missing
- A Nexus wasn't provided
- The condition wasn't clearly documented
- The VA didn't have enough information

Understanding the rules — and providing strong evidence — dramatically increases approval rates.

Putting It All Together

Myths and misunderstandings can create unnecessary fear and confusion. When you know the truth, you can make informed decisions, avoid common mistakes, and approach the VA system with confidence instead of hesitation. You've earned these benefits — and understanding the facts ensures you receive them.

In the next section, we'll wrap up the chapter by reviewing practical steps you can take to ensure you're maximizing every benefit available to you.

---

† † † † †

The VA can grant increases based on
private medical evidence alone.
You don't always need a new C&P exam
if your doctor provides clear documentation.

† † † † †

Practical Steps to Maximize Your Benefits

Maximizing your VA benefits isn't about gaming the system – it's about understanding it. When you know how the VA evaluates claims, what evidence carries the most weight, and how to stay proactive, you put yourself in the strongest possible position. These steps help you protect your rating, strengthen future claims, and ensure you're receiving every benefit available to you.

Stay Consistent with Medical Care

Regular medical treatment creates a clear record of:

- Your symptoms
- Your limitations
- How your condition changes over time

Gaps in treatment can make it harder to show worsening conditions or justify increases later.

Document Changes in Your Health

You don't need a diary – just simple notes about:

- Flare-ups
- New symptoms
- Changes in mobility
- Medication side effects
- Impact on work or daily life

These notes help you remember details during exams or when filing increases.

Use Secondary Claims Strategically

If a service-connected condition causes or worsens another condition, file a secondary claim. This is one of the most effective ways to:

- Increase your combined rating
- Recognize the full impact of your disabilities
- Strengthen your long-term support

Secondary claims are often overlooked — but they're powerful.

Request Increases When Warranted

If your condition worsens, you can request an increase. Before doing so:

- Review the rating criteria
- Gather updated medical evidence
- Consider a DBQ or Nexus letter

Don't request an increase based on a hunch — request it based on evidence.

Keep Copies of Everything

Your "*VA folder*" should include:

- All decision letters
- All medical evidence
- DBQs and Nexus letters
- Notes from appointments
- Copies of claims and appeals

This makes future claims, increases, or appeals much easier.

Stay Informed About Policy Changes

Laws and regulations change — sometimes dramatically. The PACT Act is a perfect example. Staying informed helps you:

- Identify new presumptive conditions
- Reopen old claims
- File new claims you didn't know you qualified for

A quick annual check-in with a VSO or Accredited Agent can make a big difference.

Use Accredited Representatives When Needed

VSOs, Accredited Agents, and Attorneys can:

- Spot weaknesses in your claim
- Help you gather stronger evidence
- Interpret VA language
- Guide you through appeals

You don't have to do this alone.

Putting It All Together

Maximizing your benefits isn't about doing more — it's about doing things intentionally. When you stay organized, document your symptoms, understand secondary conditions, and keep up with medical care, you build a strong foundation that supports you for years to come.

Now that we've covered how to maximize your benefits, we're ready to move into the final chapter — where we'll bring everything together and help you feel confident, prepared, and empowered as you navigate the VA system.

---

§ § § EXTRA INSIGHTS § § §

Maximizing your VA benefits isn't about squeezing the system or chasing numbers—it's about understanding the full value of what you've earned and making sure none of it goes unused. Every benefit exists because someone before you needed it, fought for it, and proved its importance. When you take the time to learn what's available and advocate for yourself, you're stepping into that same legacy of strength and persistence.

<u>INSIDER TIP</u>: *The Veterans who get the most out of the VA system aren't the ones who know every rule—they're the ones who stay curious, ask questions, and follow up when something doesn't look right. The VA is a massive organization, and sometimes the difference between "no" and "yes" is simply asking again with the right information. Keep exploring, keep learning, and keep pushing for the support that helps you live the life you've earned.*

§ § § § § § § §

Moving Forward with Confidence

The most confident Veterans weren't the ones who knew everything – they were the ones who knew where to find answers when they needed them.

VA benefits are important—but they're only one part of your life. This chapter is about perspective, planning, and peace of mind. We'll talk about what to do after your benefits are in place, how to think about future changes, and how to move forward without feeling like you're constantly bracing for the next VA letter. The goal here is simple: confidence, not chaos.

Understanding Your Rights and Responsibilities

The VA benefits system isn't just a collection of forms, ratings, and decisions — it's a set of rights you've earned through service. And like any system built on rights, it also comes with responsibilities that help keep your benefits secure and ensure the VA has the information it needs to support you.

This section brings everything into focus. It's about understanding what you're entitled to, what the VA expects from you, and how to stay empowered long after the paperwork is done.

Your Rights as a Veteran

Be Treated with Respect

Every interaction with the VA — in person, online, or by phone — should be professional and respectful. You served. You earned that.

File a Claim at Any Time

There is no deadline for filing a disability claim. Whether it's been months, years, or decades since your service, you can still file.

Submit Evidence and Be Heard

You have the right to:

- Provide medical records
- Submit lay statements
- Present new evidence
- Challenge decisions

Your voice matters in your claim.

Appeal Any Decision

If you disagree with a decision — any part of it — you have the right to appeal through multiple lanes.

Representation

You have the right to work with:

- VSOs
- Accredited agents
- Accredited attorneys

These professionals can help you navigate the process at no cost or low cost.

Privacy and Confidentiality

Your medical and personal information must be protected and handled securely.

Your Responsibilities as a Veteran

Rights come with responsibilities that help keep your benefits accurate and up to date.

Keep Your Information Current

Notify the VA if you:

- Move
- Change phone numbers
- Update your banking information
- Add or remove dependents

This prevents delays, overpayments, or missed benefits.

Attend Scheduled Exams

C&P exams are a key part of the process. Missing them can delay or jeopardize your claim.

Provide Accurate Information

Honesty is essential. Describe your symptoms truthfully — not minimized, not exaggerated.

Stay Engaged with Your Healthcare

Regular treatment helps:

- Document your condition
- Support future claims
- Protect your rating

Your medical record is one of your strongest tools.

Respond to VA Requests

If the VA asks for evidence or clarification, respond promptly. It keeps your claim moving.

Why This Matters

Understanding your rights and responsibilities gives you control. It turns the VA system from something that happens *to* you into something you can navigate with confidence. When you know what to expect — and what's expected of you — the process becomes clearer, smoother, and far less stressful.

Putting It All Together

This chapter is about empowerment. You've learned the rules, the strategies, pitfalls, and opportunities. Now you're equipped to move forward with clarity and confidence — not just in filing a claim, but in managing your benefits for the long term.

In the next section, we'll talk about building a long-term plan for your benefits, your healthcare, and your family's future — so you're not just reacting to the system but actively shaping your path.

---

† † † † †

Revisit your benefits once a year.
Life changes, conditions change,
and the VA system evolves —
staying informed keeps you empowered.

† † † † †

Building a Long-Term Plan

A VA claim isn't a one-time event — it's part of a lifelong journey. Your health may change, your family situation may shift, and new laws or benefits may become available. Building a long-term plan helps you stay ahead of these changes and ensures you're always receiving the support you've earned.

This section gives you a practical roadmap for managing your benefits over time, protecting your rating, and planning for your family's future.

Stay Engaged with Your Healthcare

Your medical record is one of your strongest tools. Over time, consistent healthcare helps:

- Document changes in your condition
- Support future increases or secondary claims
- Provide evidence for long-term stability
- Ensure you receive appropriate treatment

Even if you feel stable, annual check-ins with your providers keep your record active and accurate.

---

† † † † †

Many Veterans qualify for benefits outside the VA —
state programs, tax exemptions, education benefits, and more.
Your journey doesn't end with a rating.

† † † † †

Review Your Benefits Annually

Just like you'd review insurance or financial plans, reviewing your VA benefits once a year helps you stay informed. During your annual review, look at:

- Your current ratings
- Any new symptoms or conditions
- Changes in your family or dependents
- New laws or presumptive conditions (*like the PACT Act*)
- State-level benefits you may now qualify for

A quick meeting with a VSO or Accredited Agent can help you spot opportunities you might otherwise miss.

Plan for Future Claims or Increases

Your conditions may worsen over time — and the VA expects that. Planning ahead helps you avoid scrambling later.

Consider:

- Keeping notes about flare-ups or limitations
- Updating DBQs every few years
- Requesting increases when symptoms clearly worsen
- Filing secondary claims when new conditions develop

A proactive approach keeps your benefits aligned with your reality.

Understand Rating Protections

The VA has built-in protections that strengthen your rating over time:

- 5-year rule: Conditions are considered "*stable*"
- 10-year rule: Service connection is protected
- 20-year rule: Your rating cannot be reduced below its lowest level in the past 20 years
- 55-year rule: Routine future exams are rare after age 55

Knowing these protections helps you make informed decisions about increases or appeals.

Prepare Your Family

Your benefits don't just support you — they support your family. Preparing them now ensures they know what to do later.

Talk with your spouse or trusted family member about:

- Your ratings and conditions
- Where you keep your VA documents
- Survivor benefits like DIC
- How to contact your representative
- What to do if the VA sends a letter after your passing

A simple conversation can prevent confusion during a difficult time.

Keep Your Documents Organized

Your long-term plan should include a clear, accessible place for:

- Decision letters
- Medical records
- DBQs and Nexus letters
- Notes from appointments
- Copies of claims and appeals
- Survivor benefit information

Think of it as your "*VA binder*" — a resource your family can rely on if they ever need it.

Stay Informed About Policy Changes

VA laws evolve. New presumptive conditions are added. Exposure rules expand. Rating criteria shift. Staying informed helps you:

- Reopen old claims
- File new claims you didn't know you qualified for
- Protect your rating
- Maximize your benefits

A yearly check-in with a VSO or Accredited Agent keeps you up to date.

Putting It All Together

A long-term plan isn't complicated — it's intentional. It's about staying engaged with your healthcare, reviewing your benefits regularly, preparing your family, and keeping your documents organized. When you take these steps, you're not just navigating the VA system — you're mastering it.

Moving Forward with Confidence

The VA system can feel overwhelming at first – a maze of forms, exams, decisions, and acronyms. But by this point in the book, you've done something powerful: you've taken control of the process. You've learned how the system works, how to build strong claims, how to protect your benefits, and how to plan for the future. That knowledge is more than information – it's empowerment.

This final section of the chapter is about stepping into that confidence and carrying it with you long after the paperwork is done.

You Are Not Alone in This Process

One of the biggest misconceptions Veterans have is they must navigate the VA system by themselves. But you have:

- Accredited representatives
- VSOs
- Medical providers
- Family members
- Caregivers
- Fellow Veterans

You have a community – and you have the right to lean on it.

Your Benefits Are Earned, Not Given

It's easy to feel like you're asking for something extra when you file a claim. But you're not. You're accessing benefits that were earned through service, sacrifice, and commitment.

You're not asking for charity–You're asking for what you've earned.

That mindset shift matters.

Progress, Not Perfection

You don't have to understand everything at once. You don't have to file the perfect claim. You don't have to know every rule or regulation. What matters is progress:

- Filing the claim
- Gathering evidence
- Asking questions
- Learning the process
- Taking the next step

Every action you take moves you forward.

Your Voice Matters

Your statements, your experiences, your symptoms, your story — they matter. The VA system is built on evidence, yes, but it's also built on your lived reality.

Your voice is part of your evidence.
Your story is part of your claim.
Your truth is part of your path forward.

You Are Allowed to Advocate for Yourself

Advocacy isn't confrontation — it's clarity. It's saying:

- *"This is what I'm experiencing."*
- *"This is how it affects my life."*
- *"This is what the evidence shows."*
- *"This is what I'm entitled to."*

Advocating for yourself is not only allowed — it's necessary.

Your Future Is Bigger Than Your Claim

VA benefits are a tool, not a destination. They will help you:

- Access healthcare
- Support your family
- Maintain stability
- Plan for the future
- Live with dignity

Your claim is part of your story — but it's not the whole story.

Putting It All Together

Moving forward with confidence doesn't mean you'll never feel frustrated or uncertain. It means you now have the knowledge, tools, and support to navigate whatever comes next. You've built a foundation that will serve you for years to come — and you've done it step by step, with clarity and purpose.

With this chapter complete, you're ready to move into the next major part of the book: your Practical Tools & Guidance, where we'll shift from narrative to hands-on resources — checklists, sample letters, walkthroughs, and myth-busting sidebars designed to make the process even easier.

Practical Tools and Guidance

Even drafting a rough outline of your symptoms or timeline is progress. You can refine it later — the hardest part is getting started.

Now that you've built a strong understanding of the VA system and learned how to move forward with clarity and confidence, it's time to shift from strategy to action. The next part of this book is designed to be your toolkit — the checklists, templates, examples, and walkthroughs you can use immediately. Whether you're filing your first claim, helping someone else, or preparing for an appeal, these tools give you step-by-step support you can return to anytime.

Let's begin with one of the most helpful resources in the entire process: clear, simple checklists that guide you through filing a strong, well-organized claim from start to finish.

Checklists for Filing

A good checklist turns a complicated process into a clear, manageable series of steps. These filing checklists are designed to help you stay organized, avoid common mistakes, and make sure you're submitting the strongest claim possible. You can use them for initial claims, secondary claims, increases, or supplemental claims.

Checklist: *Initial Claim for Service Connection*

Before You File

- Confirm you have a current diagnosis
- Gather service records related to the condition
- Collect private medical records (*if applicable*)
- Write a personal statement describing your symptoms
- Identify any buddy statements you may want to include
- Review the rating criteria for your condition

Documents to Prepare

- VA Form 21-526EZ (*Application for Disability Compensation*)
    - This can also be completed online at VA.gov
- Medical records (*VA and private*)
- Service treatment records
- Nexus letter (*if needed*)
- DBQ (*if available*)
- Lay statements

Before Submitting

- Double-check that all evidence is attached
- Ensure your contact information is correct
- Save a copy of everything you submit
- Submit through VA.gov, mail, agent, or a VSO

Checklist: *Secondary Service Connection Claim*

Evidence Needed

- Diagnosis of the secondary condition
- Proof of the primary service-connected condition
- Nexus letter linking the two
- DBQ for the secondary condition
- Treatment notes showing progression

Before Submitting

- Confirm the Nexus clearly states "*at least as likely as not*"
- Attach all medical evidence
- Include a personal statement describing how the conditions interact
- Save copies of everything

Checklist: *Request for Increase*

Before You File

- Review the rating criteria for your condition
- Gather recent medical records
- Document worsening symptoms
- Consider a DBQ from your provider
- Write a personal statement describing changes

Evidence That Helps

- Updated imaging or test results
- Notes from specialists
- Medication changes
- Work impact statements
- Daily living impact statements

---

† † † † †

The VA decides based on what's written down.
If it's not documented —
by you, a buddy, or a medical provider —
it's invisible to the system.

† † † † †

Checklist: *Supplemental Claim*

Required

- New and relevant evidence
- VA Form 20-0995 (*Supplemental Claim*)

Examples of New Evidence

- Updated medical opinions
- New diagnoses
- Private medical records
- Buddy statements
- Evidence the VA previously failed to obtain

Before Submitting

- Ensure the evidence is truly new
- Confirm it directly supports the denied issue
- Attach everything in one packet if possible

---

† † † † †

Preparation isn't about paperwork —
it's about clarity.
The clearer your story,
the easier it is for the VA to understand your claim.

† † † † †

Checklist: *Preparing for a C&P Exam*

Before the Exam

- Review your symptoms
- Review your personal statement
- Bring a list of medications
- Bring mobility aids or devices you normally use
- Review the rating criteria in the 38 CFR

The Code of Federal Regulations, Title 38 (38 CFR) contains the rules the VA must follow when evaluating and deciding claims. Part 4 of this regulation—called the Schedule for Rating Disabilities—lists every ratable condition recognized by the VA and the specific criteria required for each possible rating level. These criteria outline how the VA measures symptoms, functional loss, and the impact of a condition on a Veteran's earning capacity. It can be viewed online at:

https://www.ECFR.gov/current/title-38/chapter-I/part-4

During the Exam

- Be honest and specific
- Describe your worst days, not your best
- Don't minimize symptoms
- Don't guess – say "*I'm not sure*" if needed

After the Exam

- Write down what happened
- Note any issues or concerns
- Inform your representative if something felt off

Putting It All Together

These checklists are designed to simplify the process and help you stay organized from start to finish. You can print them, save them, or use them as a quick reference whenever you're preparing a claim or appeal.

---

† † † † †

When writing a personal statement,
imagine you're explaining your condition
to someone who has never met you.
Clear, simple language beats medical jargon every time.

† † † † †

Sample Nexus Letters

A Nexus letter is a medical opinion that connects a Veteran's current disability to their military service (*or to another service-connected condition*). The VA relies heavily on these letters when deciding claims, especially when the connection isn't obvious from service records alone. They are typically obtained from your treating physician.

Below are clear, realistic, plain-language examples of Nexus letters. These are not scripts — they're templates that show the structure and medical reasoning the VA expects. To obtain and review current DBQ's, visit: **https://go.veteranrollcall.org/dbq**

NOTE: All letters should include:

- Provider's Name and Credentials
- Clinic or Practice Name
- Address
- Phone Number
- Date
- Signature

---

† † † † †

COMMON PITFALL:

Copy-and-paste statements. The VA can spot them instantly. Personalized statements carry far more weight.

† † † † †

Sample Nexus Letter #1: ***Direct Service Connection***

RE: Medical Nexus Opinion for [*Veteran's Name*]

I am a licensed [*physician/psychologist/NP/PA*] and have been treating [*Veteran's Name*] since [*date*]. I have reviewed the Veteran's medical history, service treatment records, and current symptoms.

The Veteran has a current diagnosis of [*condition*], confirmed by [*exam, imaging, testing*].

The Veteran reports that symptoms began during military service, specifically [*describe event, injury, exposure, or onset*]. This account is consistent with the medical literature and with the Veteran's documented service duties.

Medical Opinion:

Based on my review of the available records, the Veteran's history, and my medical expertise, it is at least as likely as not (50% probability or greater) that the Veteran's [*condition*] began during or is directly related to their military service.

Rationale:

- The Veteran's symptoms began during service and have continued since.
- The mechanism of injury/exposure is medically consistent with the current diagnosis.
- There is no evidence of an alternative cause that better explains the condition.

Sample Nexus Letter #2:
Secondary Service Connection

RE: Medical Nexus Opinion for [*Veteran's Name*]

I am providing a medical opinion regarding the relationship between the Veteran's service-connected [*primary condition*] and their diagnosed [*secondary condition*].

The Veteran is currently service-connected for [*primary condition*], which causes [*symptoms, limitations, gait changes, medication effects, etc.*]. The Veteran has also been diagnosed with [*secondary condition*], confirmed by [*testing, imaging, evaluation*].

Medical Opinion:

It is at least as likely as not (50% probability or greater) that the Veteran's [*secondary condition*] is caused by or aggravated by their service-connected [*primary condition*].

Rationale:

- The Veteran's altered gait due to [primary condition] places abnormal stress on [affected area], which is consistent with the development of [secondary condition].
- Medical literature supports a causal relationship between [primary condition] and [secondary condition].
- The Veteran's symptoms worsened after the progression of the primary condition, indicating aggravation.

Sample Nexus Letter #3: *Exposure-Related Condition* (*e.g., Burn Pits, Agent Orange, Gulf War*)

RE: Medical Nexus Opinion for [*Veteran's Name*]

I have reviewed the Veteran's medical history, service records, and current diagnosis of [*condition*]. The Veteran served in [*location*] during [*dates*], where they were exposed to [*burn pits, airborne hazards, Agent Orange, oil well fires, etc.*].

Medical Opinion:

It is at least as likely as not (50% probability or greater) that the Veteran's [*condition*] is related to their exposure to [*hazard*] during military service.

Rationale:

- The Veteran's exposure is consistent with known risk factors for [*condition*].
- The latency period between exposure and symptom onset is medically appropriate.
- There is no more likely alternative cause.

---

† † † † †

Most Veterans underestimate how much evidence they already have.
Medical records, emails, prescriptions, even text messages can help paint the picture.

† † † † †

Sample Nexus Letter #4: *Mental Health Condition*

RE: Medical Nexus Opinion for [*Veteran's Name*]

I am a licensed [*psychologist/psychiatrist*] and have evaluated [*Veteran's Name*] for [*condition: PTSD, depression, anxiety, etc.*].

The Veteran reports exposure to [*traumatic event*] during military service. Their symptoms — including [*list symptoms*] — are consistent with the diagnostic criteria for [*condition*].

Medical Opinion:

It is at least as likely as not (50% probability or greater) that the Veteran's [*mental health condition*] is the result of their military service.

Rationale:

- The Veteran's symptoms began after the in-service event.
- Their presentation is consistent with known responses to trauma.
- There is no evidence of a pre-service condition that better explains the symptoms.

Putting It All Together

These sample Nexus letters give Veterans and providers with a clear sense of structure, tone, and medical reasoning. They're not meant to be copied word-for-word — they're templates that show what a strong, VA-ready medical opinion looks like.

DBQ Walkthroughs

A Disability Benefits Questionnaire (DBQ) is a standardized form the VA uses to evaluate medical conditions. DBQs guide examiners through the exact criteria the VA uses to assign ratings, which makes them incredibly powerful tools for Veterans.

Understanding how a DBQ is structured helps you:

- Know what to expect during a C&P exam
- Understand how your condition is evaluated
- Identify what evidence matters most
- Communicate more clearly with your provider
- Strengthen your claim or appeal

Below is a clear, practical walkthrough of DBQs — what they include, why they matter, and how to use them effectively.

What a DBQ Is (*and isn't*)

A DBQ *is*:

- A structured medical evaluation
- A form aligned with VA rating criteria
- A tool used by VA and private providers
- Evidence that can support your claim

A DBQ *is not*:

- A guarantee of approval
- A replacement for medical records
- A place to exaggerate or minimize symptoms
- A form you must complete yourself

A DBQ is simply a medical snapshot — but a very important one.

Common Sections in Most DBQs

While each DBQ is tailored to a specific condition, most follow a similar structure. Here's what you'll typically see:

Diagnosis Section

This section confirms:

- Your current diagnosis
- The date of diagnosis
- Any related or secondary conditions

Why it matters: The VA cannot rate a condition without a confirmed diagnosis.

Medical History

This includes:

- When symptoms began
- How the condition has progressed
- Treatments you've received
- Surgeries, hospitalizations, or major events

Why it matters: This section helps establish chronicity and continuity — key elements in service connection.

Symptoms and Functional Impact

This is where the examiner documents:

- Pain levels
- Frequency of flare-ups
- Limitations in movement
- Impact on daily activities
- Impact on work

Why it matters: This section often determines your rating. The VA rates based on *functional loss*, not just diagnosis.

Range of Motion (*for musculoskeletal DBQs*)

If your condition affects joints, the examiner will measure:

- Flexion
- Extension
- Rotation
- Pain on movement
- Pain on weight-bearing
- Repetitive-use limitations

Why it matters: These measurements directly correspond to rating percentages.

Testing and Imaging

This includes:

- X-rays
- MRIs
- Lab results
- Pulmonary function tests
- Neurological exams

Why it matters: Objective findings strengthen your claim and support the examiner's conclusions.

Occupational Impact

This section asks:

- How does the condition affect your ability to work?
- Are there limitations in physical or sedentary tasks?
- Are accommodations needed?

Why it matters: This section is especially important for TDIU claims.

Medical Opinion (*if required*)

Some DBQs include a Nexus opinion section where the examiner states whether the condition is:

- At least as likely as not related to service
- Less likely than not related to service

Why it matters: This can make or break a service-connection claim.

How to Use a DBQ Effectively

Before the Exam

- Review the DBQ for your condition.
- Make notes about your symptoms and limitations.
- Bring mobility aids or devices you normally use.

During the Exam

- Be honest and specific.
- Describe your worst days, not your best.
- Don't minimize symptoms – this is not the time to "*tough it out.*"
- Don't guess; say "*I'm not sure*" if needed.

After the Exam

- Write down what happened.
- Note any issues or concerns.
- Share concerns with your representative if something felt inaccurate.

Why DBQs Matter So Much

DBQs are powerful because they:

- Align directly with rating criteria
- Provide structured medical evidence
- Reduce ambiguity in claims
- Help ensure consistency across examiners
- Can be completed by private providers (*in many cases*)

A strong DBQ can significantly strengthen your claim or appeal.

Putting It All Together

Understanding DBQs gives you a major advantage in the claims process. When you know what the examiner is looking for — and how the VA uses the information — you can approach your exam with clarity and confidence.

---

† † † † †

Templates are helpful, but your voice matters.
The strongest statements sound like
real people telling real stories —
not forms being filled out.

† † † † †

Myth-Busting Sidebars

Misinformation is one of the biggest obstacles Veterans face when navigating the VA system. These myth-busting sidebars are designed to cut through the noise and give you clear, accurate guidance. Each one addresses a common misconception and replaces it with the facts you need to make informed decisions.

Myth-Busting Sidebar #1: *"You can't file twice."*

The Myth

Some Veterans believe that once you file a claim — especially if it's denied — you can't file it again.

The Truth

You can file as many times as needed:

- New claims
- Secondary claims
- Supplemental claims
- Requests for increases
- Appeals

The VA does not limit the number of claims you can submit. What matters is whether you provide new and relevant evidence when required.

Why This Myth Exists

Older versions of the VA system were more rigid, and some Veterans were discouraged from refiling. Under the modern AMA system, refiling is normal and expected.

Myth-Busting Sidebar #2:
"VA doctors won't help."

The Myth

Some Veterans believe VA doctors are not allowed to support claims or write Nexus letters.

The Truth

VA doctors *can* help — but they are not required to write Nexus letters or DBQs. Their primary role is treatment, not claims development.

However:

- Their medical records
- Their diagnoses
- Their treatment notes
- Their documented observations

...are all powerful evidence in your claim.

Why This Myth Exists

Some VA providers decline to write Nexus letters due to workload or policy guidance. That doesn't mean they're against your claim — it simply means their role is focused on care, not documentation for compensation.

Myth-Busting Sidebar #3:
“Pension is only for the poor.”

The Myth

Many Veterans think VA pension is only for those with no income or assets.

The Truth

VA pension is needs-based, but it’s not limited to extreme poverty. Eligibility depends on:

- Wartime service
- Age or disability
- Income
- Certain allowable deductions (*like medical expenses*)

Many Veterans who assume they don’t qualify actually do – especially those with high medical costs or assisted-living expenses.

Why This Myth Exists

The term “*pension*” is often misunderstood. VA pension is a safety-net benefit, but it’s broader and more flexible than most people realize.

Bonus Sidebar:
"If I file a claim, the VA will reduce my rating."

The Myth

Veterans worry that filing anything — even a new claim — will trigger a review of all their ratings.

The Truth

Filing a new claim does not automatically trigger a review of existing ratings, though it MAY lead to your rated conditions being reviewed using newly filed medical information. The VA only re-evaluates a condition if:

- You request an increase, or
- There is clear evidence your condition has significantly improved

Most Veterans file new claims without any impact on their current ratings.

Putting It All Together

These myth-busting sidebars are designed to give you quick, confidence-building clarity. When you understand what's true — and what's not — you can make better decisions, avoid unnecessary fear, and stay focused on the evidence that matters.

---

§ § § EXTRA INSIGHTS § § §

The tools you use to navigate the VA system don't just help you stay organized—they help you stay in control. When you track your symptoms, keep copies of your records, or outline your claim story, you're doing more than managing paperwork. You're building a clear, confident foundation that supports every step of your journey. Even small habits, done consistently, can make the entire process feel less overwhelming and far more predictable.

INSIDER TIP: *VA reviewers notice when a Veteran's submission is organized, consistent, and easy to follow. A simple checklist, a folder of key documents, or a short timeline of events can quietly strengthen your claim by giving the VA a clear roadmap. You don't need fancy tools—just a system that works for you. The more clarity you create on your end, the smoother things tend to move on theirs.*

§ § § § § § § § §

Family & Caregiver Perspectives

Families often see the first signs of worsening symptoms long before the Veteran does.
Trust your instincts — your perspective is important.

The tools and guidance in the previous chapter were designed to help Veterans take control of their claims with clarity and confidence. But Veterans rarely walk this path alone. Family members, caregivers, and loved ones often play a crucial role — offering support, helping gather evidence, attending appointments, or simply being a steady presence during a stressful process.

This next chapter is dedicated to them. Whether you're a spouse, partner, parent, adult child, or close friend, your support can make a meaningful difference. The following sections will help you understand the process from your side of the table and give you practical ways to help without feeling overwhelmed.

Helping a Veteran File

Supporting a Veteran through the VA claims process can feel intimidating at first — especially if you're not familiar with the terminology, the forms, or the steps involved. But your role doesn't require you to be an expert. What matters most is your presence, your patience, and your ability to help the Veteran stay organized and supported.

This section gives you clear, practical ways to help a Veteran file a claim while respecting their autonomy and comfort level.

Understanding Your Role

Family members and caregivers often help Veterans by:

- Gathering documents
- Keeping track of deadlines
- Helping describe symptoms or changes
- Providing emotional support
- Attending appointments
- Helping communicate with representatives

You don't need to speak for the Veteran — you simply help them stay steady and organized.

How You Can Help Before Filing

Create a Calm, Supportive Environment

Filing a claim can bring up old memories, frustrations, or anxieties. Your steady presence helps the Veteran feel grounded.

Help Gather Key Documents

You can assist by locating:

- Service records
- Medical records
- Decision letters
- Notes about symptoms
- Past claims or appeals

Having everything in one place reduces stress and confusion.

Encourage the Veteran to Describe Their Symptoms Honestly

Many Veterans minimize their struggles. You can gently remind them:

- *"Tell them what it's like on your worst days."*
- *"It's okay to be honest — this is about getting support."*

Your perspective can help them articulate things they may overlook.

How You Can Help During the Filing Process

Assist With Online Navigation

VA.gov can be confusing. You can help by:

- Navigating the website
- Uploading documents
- Double-checking forms
- Saving copies of submissions

You're not filing *for* them — you're helping them stay organized.

Attend Appointments (*If the Veteran Wants You There*)

Your presence can help the Veteran:

- Remember details
- Stay calm
- Feel supported

You can also provide observations if the examiner asks, but only with the Veteran's permission.

Help Track Deadlines

The VA system has strict timelines. You can help by:

- Marking calendars
- Setting reminders
- Keeping a simple checklist

This prevents missed opportunities or delays.

How You Can Help After Filing

Watch for VA Letters or Emails

Sometimes Veterans miss important notices. You can help by:

- Checking mail together
- Reviewing VA.gov updates
- Keeping copies of everything

Support the Veteran Emotionally

Waiting for a decision can be stressful. Your encouragement matters more than you may realize.

Help Prepare for C&P Exams

You can:

- Review symptoms together
- Help the Veteran recall examples
- Remind them to be honest and specific

Your perspective can help them articulate daily challenges.

What You Should *Not* Do

Don't Speak Over the Veteran

Your role is supportive, not authoritative. The VA needs to hear the Veteran's voice.

Don't Pressure Them

Filing can be emotional. Move at a pace that feels comfortable for the Veteran.

Don't Guess or Exaggerate

Accuracy is essential. Stick to what you know and have observed.

Your Support Makes a Difference

You don't need to know the regulations or memorize the forms. Your presence, organization, and encouragement can make the entire process smoother and less overwhelming. Veterans often carry the weight of their experiences quietly — having someone walk beside them can make all the difference.

Helping a Veteran file a claim is one of the most meaningful ways a family member or caregiver can offer support. But your role doesn't end there. Families also need to understand what benefits may be available *to them* — especially in the event of a Veteran's passing. Survivor benefits can provide stability, healthcare, and financial support during one of the most difficult times a family can face. In the next section, we'll walk through these benefits clearly and compassionately, so you know exactly what support exists and how to access it.

Understanding Survivor Benefits

Survivor benefits are among the most important – and often least understood – parts of the VA system. These benefits exist to ensure that when a Veteran passes away, their family is not left without support. Whether you're a spouse, partner, dependent child, or caregiver, understanding these benefits now can prevent confusion and stress later.

This section explains the major survivor benefits in clear, practical terms, so families know what they may qualify for and how to prepare.

Dependency and Indemnity Compensation (DIC)

DIC is the cornerstone of VA survivor benefits. It is a tax-free monthly payment made to eligible survivors of:

- Veterans who died from a service-connected condition
- Veterans who were rated totally disabled (*100% or TDIU*) for a qualifying period before death
- Service members who died on active duty

DIC is one of the most significant benefits available to surviving spouses and dependents.

Who Is Eligible for DIC?

Surviving Spouses

A spouse may qualify if:

- The Veteran's death was caused by a service-connected condition, or
- The Veteran was rated totally disabled for:
    - 10 years before death, or
    - 5 years from discharge to death, or
    - 1 year if the Veteran was a former POW

Spouses may also qualify if they:

- Lived with the Veteran continuously until death (*with some exceptions*)
- Remarried after age 57 (*and in some cases after age 55*)

Dependent Children

Children may qualify if they are:

- Under age 18
- Between 18–23 and attending school
- Permanently incapable of self-support due to disability

Dependent Parents

Parents with financial need may qualify for Parents' DIC.

CHAMPVA (*Healthcare for Survivors*)

CHAMPVA provides healthcare coverage for eligible surviving spouses and dependents if the Veteran was:

- Rated permanently and totally disabled, or
- Passed away from a service-connected condition

CHAMPVA can be used with Medicare, private insurance, or as a standalone program.

Survivors' and Dependents' Educational Assistance (DEA)

DEA provides education benefits for spouses and children, including:

- College
- Technical or vocational training
- Apprenticeships
- Career programs

This benefit can be life-changing for families planning long-term stability.

Burial and Memorial Benefits

The VA offers several forms of support to honor the Veteran's service:

- Burial allowances
- Headstones or markers
- Presidential Memorial Certificates
- Burial in a VA national cemetery

These benefits help families during a difficult and emotional time.

Accrued Benefits

If the Veteran was owed benefits at the time of death — such as a pending claim or unpaid compensation — eligible survivors may receive those funds.

This includes:

- Claims still in progress
- Retroactive payments
- Unpaid monthly benefits

Survivor Pension

For low-income surviving spouses and children of wartime Veterans, the VA offers a needs-based pension. This benefit can be especially helpful when combined with:

- Medical expense deductions
- Assisted-living costs
- In-home care expenses

Many families qualify without realizing it.

Preparing Ahead: *What Families Should Know*

Understanding survivor benefits now can prevent confusion later. Families should:

- Know the Veteran's ratings and conditions
- Keep copies of decision letters and medical records
- Understand the basics of DIC eligibility
- Know where important documents are stored
- Have access to VA.gov login information (*if appropriate*)
- Know how to contact the Veteran's representative

A simple conversation today can save months of stress later.

Putting It All Together

Survivor benefits exist to protect families when they need support the most. Whether it's monthly compensation, healthcare, education assistance, or burial benefits, these programs honor the Veteran's service by caring for the people they loved. Understanding these benefits now ensures families are prepared, informed, and supported — no matter what the future holds.

---

† † † † †

Don't forget your own well-being.
Supporting a Veteran is meaningful work,
but you deserve rest, support, and space too.

† † † † †

Estate Planning & VA Benefits

Estate planning isn't just about finances – it's about clarity, security, and making sure your wishes are honored. For Veterans and their families, VA benefits play a unique role in this process. Understanding how these benefits interact with wills, trusts, long-term care, and end-of-life planning can help families avoid confusion and ensure everything is handled smoothly.

This section breaks down the essentials in simple, practical terms.

Why Estate Planning Matters for Veterans

Estate planning helps ensure:

- Your wishes are followed
- Your family knows what to do
- Important documents are easy to find
- Benefits continue without interruption
- Stress is reduced during difficult times

For Veterans, estate planning also helps protect:

- Survivor benefits
- Pension eligibility
- Long-term care options
- Access to healthcare programs like CHAMPVA

Key Documents Every Veteran Should Have

These documents form the foundation of a solid estate plan:

Last Will and Testament

Specifies:

- How your assets are distributed
- Who manages your estate
- Guardianship for minor children

Durable Power of Attorney

Allows someone you trust to handle:

- Financial decisions
- VA paperwork
- Banking and bills

This is especially important if you become unable to manage your affairs.

Healthcare Power of Attorney

Designates someone to make medical decisions if you cannot.

Advance Healthcare Directive (*Living Will*)

Outlines your wishes for:

- Life-sustaining treatment
- End-of-life care
- Medical interventions

VA-Specific Documents

These may include:

- DD-214 (*always keep multiple copies*)
- VA award letters
- Rating decisions
- List of service-connected conditions
- VA.gov login information (*shared only with trusted individuals*)

Having these documents organized and accessible is a tremendous gift to your family.

How VA Benefits Fit into Estate Planning

VA benefits interact with estate planning in several important ways:

DIC Eligibility Depends on Documentation

Surviving spouses often need:

- The Veteran's rating history
- Evidence of service-connected conditions
- Copies of decision letters
- Medical records

If these documents are missing, DIC claims can be delayed.

Pension Eligibility Can Be Affected by Assets

VA pension is needs-based. Estate planning can help families:

- Understand allowable medical deductions
- Plan for assisted-living or in-home care
- Avoid unintentional disqualification

A financial planner familiar with VA rules can be extremely helpful.

Long-Term Care Planning

VA benefits may help cover:

- In-home care
- Assisted living
- Nursing home care
- Adult day programs

But these benefits often require:

- Documentation of medical need
- Proof of income and assets
- Evidence of service-connected conditions

Planning ahead prevents gaps in care.

Protecting CHAMPVA Eligibility

Surviving spouses and dependents may qualify for CHAMPVA if:

- The Veteran was permanently and totally disabled, or
- The Veteran passed away from a service-connected condition

Estate planning ensures families know how to maintain eligibility.

Ensuring Smooth Access to VA.gov and eBenefits

Families often struggle to access:

- Pending claims
- Decision letters
- Payment information

A simple list of:

- Login credentials
- Representatives' contact information
- Important VA documents

...can prevent major delays.

Practical Steps Families Can Take Now

Create a "*VA Binder*"

Include:

- DD-214
- Rating decisions
- Medical records
- Survivor benefit information
- Contact info for representatives

Have a Family Conversation

Discuss:

- Wishes for care
- Important documents
- Who will handle VA matters
- Where everything is stored

Review Benefits Annually

Laws change. Ratings change. Family needs change.

Consult Professionals When Needed

Consider:

- Estate planning attorneys
- Financial planners familiar with VA rules
- Accredited VA representatives

Putting It All Together

Estate planning isn't about fear — it's about preparation. When Veterans and families understand how VA benefits fit into the bigger picture, they gain peace of mind and confidence. A little planning today can prevent confusion, delays, and stress tomorrow.

---

† † † † †

Surviving spouses may qualify for benefits even if the Veteran never filed a claim during their lifetime. It's worth exploring every option.

† † † † †

Emotional Support During the Process

The VA claims process isn't just paperwork – it's personal. For many Veterans, filing a claim means revisiting painful memories, acknowledging limitations, or confronting experiences they've tried to bury. For families and caregivers, supporting a Veteran through this process can be both meaningful and emotionally challenging.

This section offers practical, compassionate guidance to help you support the Veteran you care about while also taking care of yourself.

Understanding the Emotional Landscape

Veterans may experience a wide range of emotions during the claims process:

- Frustration
- Anxiety
- Shame or guilt
- Anger
- Avoidance
- Fear of being judged
- Fear of being denied

These reactions are normal. The process can stir up old wounds, challenge a Veteran's sense of identity, or bring back memories they've worked hard to suppress.

Your understanding and patience can make a profound difference.

How to Support a Veteran Emotionally

Listen Without Fixing

Veterans often need space to talk through their experiences. You don't need to solve the problem — just listening with empathy can be incredibly grounding.

Validate Their Feelings

Simple phrases like:

- *"That makes sense."*
- *"I hear you."*
- *"That sounds really difficult."*

...can help the Veteran feel understood and supported.

Encourage, Don't Push

Some days the Veteran may feel ready to tackle paperwork. Other days, they may need space. Encouragement works better than pressure.

Celebrate Small Wins

Submitting a form, attending an appointment, or gathering records are all meaningful steps. Recognizing progress helps maintain momentum.

Be Present During Difficult Moments

C&P exams, retelling traumatic events, or reading decision letters can be emotionally heavy. Your presence — even silent — can be a source of strength.

Supporting Yourself as a Caregiver or Family Member

Caring for a Veteran can be deeply rewarding, but it can also be emotionally draining. Your well-being matters too.

Set Healthy Boundaries

It's okay to say:

- *"I need a moment."*
- *"Let's take a break."*
- *"Can we come back to this later?"*

Supporting doesn't mean sacrificing your own emotional health.

Seek Support When Needed

Talking to:

- Friends
- Family
- Support groups
- Counselors

...can help you process your own feelings.

Recognize Your Limits

You're not expected to be a therapist, legal expert, or medical professional. Your role is support — not perfection.

Practice Self-Care

You can't pour from an empty cup. Even small acts matter:

- A walk
- A quiet moment
- A hobby
- Rest
- Time with loved ones

Navigating Tough Conversations

Some conversations may be difficult, especially when discussing:

- Trauma
- Declining health
- Financial stress
- Survivor benefits
- End-of-life planning

Approach these topics gently, with compassion and patience. It's okay to take breaks, revisit topics later, or seek professional guidance.

When to Encourage Professional Help

If the Veteran shows signs of:

- Severe depression
- Withdrawal
- Anger that feels unmanageable
- Difficulty coping
- Emotional numbness
- Thoughts of self-harm

...it may be time to encourage them to speak with a mental health professional or someone they trust. You don't have to handle these moments alone.

Putting It All Together

Supporting a Veteran through the VA process is an act of love, patience, and resilience. Your presence matters. Your encouragement matters. Your understanding matters. And taking care of yourself matters just as much.

This chapter has given you the tools to support the Veteran you care about — practically, emotionally, and compassionately. Together, you can navigate the challenges, celebrate the victories, and move forward with confidence and connection.

---

† † † † †

Caregivers can submit their own statements to the VA.
A short, honest description of what you see
day-to-day can make a real difference.

† † † † †

Bringing It Together: *Stories, Lessons, Next Steps*

Sharing your experience with another Veteran can help them start their own journey — and reinforce what you've learned along the way.

You've learned how the VA system works, how to build strong claims, how to support a Veteran, and how to plan for the future. Now it's time to step back and look at the bigger picture — the real-world impact of these benefits, the lessons learned from others who've walked this path, and the resources that can help you keep moving forward. This final chapter brings together stories, insights, and practical next steps to leave you confident, prepared, and supported as you continue your journey

Real-World Success Stories (*Anonymized*)

Sometimes the best way to understand the VA process is to see how it plays out in real life. These brief, anonymized stories highlight different types of claims — initial, secondary, and appeals — and show how Veterans successfully navigated the system using the same tools and strategies you've learned in this book.

Each story is simple, honest, and focused on what made the difference.

---

† † † † †

The most powerful stories aren't
the ones with perfect records —
they're the ones told with
honesty, courage, and persistence.

† † † † †

Success Story #1:
Initial Claim That Finally Connected the Dots

Background:
A Veteran in his early 40s had chronic knee pain that began during service but never received a formal diagnosis while enlisted. He assumed he "*didn't have enough proof*" to file.

What Changed:

He gathered:

- A current diagnosis from his doctor
- A personal statement describing years of pain
- A buddy statement from a former teammate who remembered the injury
- Service records showing repeated physical training and field exercises

Outcome:
The VA granted service connection at 20%. The key was not a single "*smoking gun,*" but a combination of consistent evidence that told a clear story.

Lesson:
You don't need perfect records — you need a clear, credible connection.

Success Story #2: *Secondary Claim That Made All the Difference*

Background:
A Veteran with a service-connected ankle injury developed hip and lower-back pain over time. He didn't realize these could be connected.

What Changed:

His provider wrote a Nexus letter explaining how his altered gait caused additional strain on his hip and back. A DBQ documented limited range of motion and pain.

Outcome:
The VA granted secondary service connection for both conditions, increasing his overall rating significantly.

Lesson:
Secondary conditions are often overlooked — but they can be life-changing.

---

† † † † †

COMMON PITFALL:

Ignoring VA letters because they look confusing.
Some letters require action —
missing a deadline can stall your claim.

† † † † †

Success Story #3:
Appeal That Turned a Denial into a Win

Background:
A Veteran filed for migraines but was denied due to "*insufficient evidence*." She almost gave up.

What Changed:

She filed a Supplemental Claim with:

- A new neurologist's opinion
- A detailed headache log
- Updated imaging
- A personal statement describing the impact on work

Outcome:
Her claim was approved at 50% on appeal.

Lesson:
A denial isn't the end — it's often just the beginning of a stronger claim.

Success Story #4:
Family Found Stability Through Survivor Benefits

Background:
A surviving spouse wasn't sure she qualified for DIC after her husband passed away from a heart condition.

What Changed:

A VSO reviewed his records and discovered the Veteran had been rated 100% for more than 10 years.

Outcome:
She qualified for DIC, CHAMPVA, and educational benefits for her children.

Lesson:
Families often qualify for more than they realize — and help is available.

Putting It All Together

These stories show that success doesn't come from luck — it comes from clarity, evidence, persistence, and support. Every Veteran's path is different, but the principles remain the same: stay organized, stay honest, stay informed, and don't give up.

Lessons Learned from Common Mistakes

The success stories in the previous section show what's possible when a claim is built with clarity, evidence, and persistence. But just as important as knowing what works is understanding what *doesn't.* Many Veterans run into the same avoidable pitfalls — not because they did anything wrong, but because the VA system is complex and often confusing. In the next section, we'll break down the most common mistakes Veterans make, and the lessons learned from each, so you can move forward with confidence and avoid unnecessary setbacks.

Even the most prepared Veterans can stumble during the claims process. The good news is that most mistakes are easy to avoid once you know what to look for. This section highlights the most common issues Veterans face — and the simple lessons that can help you stay on track.

Mistake #1: *Filing Without a Current Diagnosis*

The Issue

A Veteran submits a claim for a condition they experience but haven't had formally diagnosed.

Why It Matters

The VA cannot grant service connection without a current, documented diagnosis.

Lesson Learned

Before filing, make sure you have a clear diagnosis from a qualified medical provider. Symptoms alone aren't enough — the VA needs a medical label to work with.

Mistake #2: *Minimizing Symptoms During Exams*

The Issue

Veterans often "*tough it out*" during C&P exams, downplaying pain or limitations.

Why It Matters

The VA rates are based on functional loss — what you can and *cannot* do.

Lesson Learned

Describe your worst days, not your best. Honesty is not complaining — it's essential.

Mistake #3: *Assuming the VA Will Gather All Evidence*

The Issue

Veterans believe the VA will automatically collect every record needed.

Why It Matters

The VA tries, but records can be missed, incomplete, or unavailable.

Lesson Learned

Submit your own copies of medical records, private treatment notes, and supporting documents. Don't rely on the VA to find everything.

Mistake #4: *Not Reading Decision Letters Carefully*

The Issue

Veterans skim decision letters and miss key details about why a claim was denied.

Why It Matters

The denial reason tells you exactly what evidence is missing.

Lesson Learned

Read every decision letter slowly and highlight:

- The VA's reasoning
- What evidence they considered
- What evidence they didn't have
- What they say is missing

This becomes your roadmap for the next step.

Mistake #5: *Waiting Too Long to Appeal*

The Issue

Veterans miss appeal deadlines because they feel discouraged or confused.

Why It Matters

Appeal windows are strict. Missing one can reset the entire process.

Lesson Learned

Mark deadlines on a calendar. If you're unsure what to do, talk to a VSO or Accredited Agent immediately.

Mistake #6: *Not Considering Secondary Conditions*

The Issue

Veterans file only for their primary condition and overlook related issues.

Why It Matters

Secondary conditions can significantly increase your overall rating and improve quality of life.

Lesson Learned

If a service-connected condition causes or worsens another condition, file for it. Secondary claims are powerful and often overlooked.

Mistake #7: *Submitting Claims Without Personal Statements*

The Issue

Veterans rely solely on medical records.

Why It Matters

Your personal statement explains how the condition affects your daily life — something medical records often miss.

Lesson Learned

A clear, honest personal statement strengthens your claim and gives context to your symptoms.

Mistake #8: *Giving Up After a Denial*

The Issue

A Veteran receives a denial and assumes the process is over.

Why It Matters

Many denials are fixable with new evidence or a clearer explanation.

Lesson Learned

A denial is not a verdict — it's feedback. Use it to build a stronger claim.

Mistake #9: *Not Asking for Help*

The Issue

Veterans try to navigate the system alone.

Why It Matters

VSOs and accredited agents exist for a reason — they know the system inside and out.

Lesson Learned

You don't have to do this alone. Support is available, free, and effective.

Mistake #10: *Not Keeping Copies of Everything*

The Issue

Documents get lost, overwritten, or forgotten.

Why It Matters

Having your own copies protects you if something goes missing.

Lesson Learned

Create a simple "*VA folder*" — digital or physical — and save every form, letter, and record.

Putting It All Together

These lessons aren't about blame — they're about empowerment. When you understand the common pitfalls, you can avoid them, stay organized, and move through the process with confidence. Every Veteran deserves a fair, accurate decision, and these insights help you get there.

---

† † † † †

Many successful claims and appeals come from
Veterans who simply didn't give up.
Persistence is often the deciding factor.

† † † † †

The Impact on Families

VA benefits are often described in terms of percentages, ratings, and compensation tables — but their true impact is far more personal. When a Veteran receives the support they've earned, the entire family feels the difference. These brief, anonymized stories highlight how benefits can transform daily life, strengthen relationships, and provide long-term security.

These aren't dramatic tales — they're real, everyday moments that show why this process matters.

Family Story #1: *Stability After Years of Uncertainty*

A Veteran in his 50s had been struggling with chronic back pain for decades. His wife had watched him push through work, miss family events, and hide his discomfort. When he finally filed a claim and received a fair rating, something shifted.

What changed for the family:

- They no longer had to choose between medical bills and household expenses
- The Veteran felt validated — his pain was finally acknowledged
- His wife said she "*got her husband back*" because he no longer felt he had to suffer in silence

Impact: Financial stability brought emotional stability. The entire household felt lighter.

Family Story #2: *A Child's Future Made Possible*

A surviving spouse with two young children wasn't sure how she would afford college for them after her husband passed away. She didn't know she qualified for DIC or educational benefits.

With help from a VSO, she applied and was approved.

What changed for the family:

- Monthly DIC payments provided steady support
- DEA benefits opened the door to college for her children
- CHAMPVA ensured they had reliable healthcare

Impact: Her children's futures expanded from uncertainty to opportunity.

Family Story #3: *Relief for a Caregiver Who Had Been Carrying the Load Alone*

A Veteran with PTSD had difficulty navigating the claims process. His adult daughter stepped in to help — gathering records, attending appointments, and offering emotional support.

When his claim was approved, she said:

"It wasn't just the money. It was seeing him finally get the help he deserved."

What changed for the family:

- The Veteran began receiving consistent treatment
- The daughter felt less alone in supporting him
- The family had access to resources they didn't know existed

Impact: The approval brought not just financial relief, but emotional healing.

Family Story #4: *A Veteran Who Finally Asked for Help — and How It Changed Everything*

A Veteran who had always been the "*strong one*" resisted filing a claim. His spouse gently encouraged him, reminding him that asking for help wasn't weakness.

When he finally filed and received benefits:

What changed for the family:

- The Veteran felt seen and supported
- His spouse felt relieved that he was finally getting care
- Their relationship strengthened because they faced the process together

Impact: The claim became a turning point — not just financially, but emotionally.

Why These Stories Matter

These stories show that VA benefits aren't just numbers on a page. They're:

- A child's education
- A spouse's peace of mind
- A caregiver's relief
- A Veteran's dignity
- A family's stability
- A future that feels possible again

When a Veteran receives the benefits they've earned, the entire family moves forward together.

Where to Get Help: *VSOs, Accredited Agents, and State Offices*

The stories in the previous section show just how deeply VA benefits can shape the lives of Veterans and their families. But no one has to navigate this system alone. There are trained professionals — free, accredited, and ready to help — who understand the process and can guide you every step of the way. In the next section, we'll look at the organizations and individuals who can support you, how to find them, and what to expect when you work with them.

The VA system can feel overwhelming, but you don't have to go through it by yourself. There are dedicated professionals whose entire mission is to help Veterans and families navigate claims, appeals, and benefits. This section explains who they are, what they do, and how to find the right support for your needs.

Veterans Service Organizations (VSOs)

VSOs are nonprofit organizations that provide free assistance to Veterans and families. They are often the first stop for many people because they combine experience, training, and a deep understanding of the VA system.

What VSOs Can Help With

- Filing initial claims
- Gathering evidence
- Writing statements
- Preparing appeals
- Understanding decision letters
- Accessing survivor benefits

Examples of Well-Known VSOs

- American Legion – ***https://www.legion.org***
- Disabled American Veterans (DAV) – ***https://www.dav.org***
- Veterans of Foreign Wars (VFW) – ***https://www.vfw.org***
- AMVETS – ***https://www.amvets.org***
- Paralyzed Veterans of America (PVA) – ***https://pva.org***

Why VSOs Matter

VSOs are trusted, experienced, and free. They work with thousands of Veterans every year and understand the system inside and out.

Accredited Agents

Accredited agents are trained professionals authorized by the VA to assist with claims and appeals. They must pass exams, complete ongoing training, and follow strict ethical guidelines.

What Accredited Agents Can Do

- Help develop strong claims
- Review medical evidence
- Assist with complex appeals
- Provide personalized guidance
- Represent you before the VA

Why Many Veterans Choose Accredited Agents

- They often specialize in specific types of claims
- They may offer more individualized attention
- They can help with higher-level appeals

Important Note

Accredited agents may charge fees only after a decision is made and <u>only</u> for appeal-related work. Initial claims must always be free.

State Veterans' Affairs Offices

Every state has its own Veterans Affairs department, separate from the federal VA. These offices offer powerful resources that many Veterans don't realize exist.

What State Offices Provide

- State-specific benefits (*tax breaks, tuition, hunting/fishing licenses, etc.*)
- Help with federal VA claims
- Access to state Veterans homes
- Local outreach programs
- In-person assistance

Why State Offices Are Valuable

State benefits vary widely — and some are extremely generous. A quick visit to your state's Veterans Affairs website can reveal benefits you didn't know you qualified for.

---

† † † † †

Next steps don't always mean more paperwork.
Sometimes the next step is simply understanding
your benefits and living your life with confidence.

† † † † †

How to Choose the Right Support

Choosing between a VSO, accredited agent, or state office depends on your needs.

Choose a VSO if you want:

- Free, accessible support
- Help with initial claims
- A local representative

Choose an Accredited Agent if you want:

- Help with complex appeals
- Specialized knowledge
- More personalized attention

Choose a State Office if you want:

- Access to state-specific benefits
- Local programs and resources
- In-person help close to home

There's no wrong choice — only the choice that fits your situation best.

What to Expect When Working with a Representative

They will review your records.

Expect them to ask for decision letters, medical records, and service documents.

They will help you understand your options.

They'll explain whether you should file a new claim, a supplemental claim, or an appeal.

They will help you stay organized.

Representatives know what evidence matters and how to present it clearly.

They will advocate for you.

They can communicate with the VA on your behalf and help you respond to requests.

They will keep your information confidential.

Accredited representatives follow strict privacy and ethical rules.

Putting It All Together

You don't have to navigate the VA system alone. Whether you choose a VSO, an accredited agent, or your state Veterans office, support is available – free, experienced, and ready to help. These professionals can guide you through the process, strengthen your claim, and give you the confidence that you're not walking this path by yourself.

Tools You Can Use Today

Now that you know where to find trusted support — from VSOs to accredited agents to state offices — it's helpful to have a set of tools you can use on your own, anytime. The VA has made major improvements to its online systems, and there are hotlines, portals, and state resources designed to make the process easier. In the next section, you'll find a curated list of tools you can use today to check your benefits, upload evidence, track claims, and get help when you need it.

The VA system can feel complex, but there are powerful tools available to help you stay informed, organized, and supported. These resources are free, accessible, and designed to make navigating benefits easier for Veterans and families.

Below is a practical, easy-to-use list of tools you can rely on right now.

VA.gov — Your Central Hub

VA.gov is the primary online portal for Veterans and families. It's the fastest way to:

- File a claim
- Upload evidence
- Track claim status
- View decision letters
- Manage healthcare appointments
- Refill prescriptions
- Update direct deposit information
- Access survivor benefits

Why it matters: Everything is in one place, and the system has become far more user-friendly in recent years.

VA Health and Benefits Mobile App

The official VA app allows you to:

- View disability ratings
- Access digital VA ID cards
- Check claim status
- Message your healthcare team
- Refill medications
- Upload documents

Why it matters: It puts your benefits in your pocket – no computer required.

---

eBenefits (Legacy Portal)

While VA.gov has replaced most functions, eBenefits still offers:

- Certificate of Eligibility (COE) for VA home loans
- Some historical claim information
- Access to older documents

Why it matters: It is still useful for certain tasks, especially home loan benefits.

VA Hotlines You Can Call Today

These hotlines connect you directly with VA staff who can answer questions, provide support, or help you navigate benefits.

VA Benefits Hotline

For questions about claims, compensation, pension, and appeals.

VA Health Care Hotline

For healthcare enrollment, appointments, and medical questions.

Caregiver Support Line

For caregivers needing guidance, resources, or emotional support.

Veterans Crisis Line

For immediate support during emotional distress — available 24/7.

Why it matters: Sometimes talking to a real person is the fastest way to get clarity.

---

† † † † †

COMMON PITFALL:

Thinking you have to remember every detail
of your service or medical history.
You don't — you just need to tell your story consistently.

† † † † †

State Veterans Affairs Websites

Every state offers its own benefits, which may include:

- Property tax exemptions
- Tuition waivers
- State Veterans homes
- Hunting and fishing licenses
- Employment programs
- State-specific disability benefits

Why it matters: State benefits can be incredibly valuable — and many Veterans do not know they exist.

National Resource Directory

A comprehensive database of:

- Community programs
- Nonprofit services
- Housing resources
- Employment support
- Caregiver programs

Why it matters: It connects Veterans and families to thousands of vetted resources nationwide.

Vet Centers

Vet Centers offer confidential counseling and support for:

- PTSD
- Combat stress
- Military sexual trauma
- Family counseling
- Transition support

Why it matters: Vet Centers provide a safe, private space for Veterans and families — no cost, no judgment.

MyHealtheVet

A secure portal for managing VA healthcare:

- View lab results
- Send secure messages
- Refill prescriptions
- Access medical records

Why it matters: It keeps your healthcare organized and accessible.

Putting It All Together

These tools give you the power to take control of your benefits, stay informed, and get help when you need it. Whether you're filing a claim, supporting a Veteran, or planning for the future, these resources make the process clearer, faster, and more manageable.

Final Encouragement

You now have the tools, knowledge, and resources to navigate the VA system with confidence. You've seen real-world examples, learned from common mistakes, explored the impact on families, and discovered where to find support when you need it. The final step is not about forms or evidence — it's about you. This closing message is here to remind you of your strength, your service, and your right to be supported as you move forward.

You've reached the end of this guide, but not the end of your journey. Whether you're a Veteran, a spouse, a caregiver, or a family member, you've taken an important step simply by seeking clarity and understanding. The VA system can be complex, but you've shown determination, patience, and courage — the same qualities that carried you through service, through challenges, and through life.

This final message is here to remind you of a few truths that matter more than any form or rating.

You Are Not Alone

No Veteran walks this path alone — not truly. There are people ready to help:

- VSOs
- Accredited agents
- State offices
- Healthcare providers
- Family
- Friends
- Fellow Veterans

Support is not a sign of weakness. It's a sign of wisdom.

Your Service Matters

Your experiences, your sacrifices, your injuries — seen and unseen — matter. You earned these benefits through service to your country. Filing a claim is not asking for a favor. It's accessing what you've earned.

You deserve care.

You deserve support.

You deserve recognition.

Your Story Has Power

The VA system runs on evidence, but it also runs on your voice. Your story — your symptoms, your struggles, your daily challenges — is part of the truth the VA needs to hear.

You don't have to be perfect.

You don't have to remember every detail.

You just have to be honest.

Your truth is enough.

Progress Is Still Progress

Some days will feel easy. Some will feel heavy. Some will feel like you're moving forward, and others like you're standing still. But every step counts:

- Gathering a document
- Writing a statement
- Attending an appointment
- Asking for help
- Filing a claim
- Filing an appeal

Progress is progress — no matter how small.

Your Family Is Part of This Journey

If you're a family member or caregiver reading this, know this:

Your support matters.

Your patience matters.

Your presence matters.

You are part of the Veteran's strength, and your well-being is just as important.

The Future Is Bigger Than the Process

VA benefits are not the destination — they're a foundation. They help Veterans:

- Heal
- Stabilize
- Plan
- Grow
- Support their families
- Build the next chapter of their lives

This book has given you the tools to navigate the system, but the real story is what comes after: stability, relief, opportunities, and the peace of mind that benefits can bring.

A Final Word

If you take nothing else from this book, take this:

You are worthy of support.

You are worthy of care.

You are worthy of the benefits you earned.

And you are capable — fully capable — of navigating this system with confidence, clarity, and strength.

This isn't the end.

It's the beginning of a more informed, empowered, supported chapter of your life.

---

§ § § EXTRA INSIGHTS § § §

When you step back and look at the entire VA process, it's easy to feel like the pieces are scattered—claims, evidence, exams, decisions, appeals. But here's the truth: once you understand how those pieces fit, the system becomes far less intimidating. Every form you complete, every record you gather, every step you take adds clarity to your story and strengthens your path forward. Progress doesn't always feel dramatic, but it builds quietly, one decision at a time.

INSIDER TIP: *VA reviewers don't expect perfection—they expect consistency. When your claim, your evidence, and your explanations all point in the same direction, you create a narrative that's hard to ignore. Bringing everything together isn't just the final step; it's the moment your work starts speaking for you.*

§ § § § § § § § §

Epilogue

You're Not Done — You're Just Beginning

If you've made it to this point, take a moment — seriously — and breathe. You've walked through a system that confuses millions of people. You've learned the rules, the language, the shortcuts, and the pitfalls. You've gained clarity where there was once frustration, and confidence where there was once doubt.

Whether you're a Veteran, a spouse, a caregiver, or someone simply trying to help, you've taken steps that will make a real difference in someone's life — maybe even your own.

The VA system isn't perfect. It's slow, it's complex, and it can test your patience. But it also exists for a reason: to support those who served, those who sacrificed, and those who stood beside them. You are part of that story now.

As you move forward, remember:

- You don't have to know everything — just where to find answers.
- You don't have to do everything — just take the next step.
- You don't have to walk alone — support is out there.

Your journey doesn't end with a decision letter. It continues with the stability, clarity, and confidence you've gained along the way. And if you ever feel lost again, come back to these pages. They'll be here — steady, clear, and ready to guide you.

You've earned your benefits
You've earned your peace of mind
You've earned the right to move forward with certainty.

Thank you for letting me walk this path with you.

§ § § EXTRA INSIGHTS § § §

A Final Word for the Road Ahead: *You've just taken the time to understand a system that wasn't built to be simple, yet you stayed with it, page after page, determined to make sense of what matters for your future. That alone says something powerful about you. The path forward may still have twists, but you now carry the clarity, tools, and confidence to navigate it with purpose.*

Every step you take—whether it's filing a claim, asking a question, or simply learning something new—moves you closer to the support you've earned. Keep going. Keep asking. Keep advocating for yourself and your family. You've already proven you're capable of more than you realized. The next chapter of your journey isn't written yet, but you're walking into it stronger, wiser, and far from alone.

§ § § § § § § §

Acknowledgements

Writing this next book has reminded me once again that no meaningful work is ever done alone. It would not be possible without the impact of those who show up — with honesty, encouragement, and the occasional reality check.

To my wife, **Kristen**. She sees every chapter before anyone else and ensures my ramblings become something clear and useful. Her insight, patience, and heart help make these books truly uplifting for Veterans and their families.

To **Rob Clark**, a former teammate at Nucor and a man whose dedication to Veterans is matched only by his ability to make hard work look effortless. Through Operation Steel Warrior and his partnership with the Gary Sinise Foundation, Rob continues to change lives in meaningful ways. I sincerely appreciate his willingness to review this book and provide valuable feedback to improve the message.

To **Tony Cox**, who has been beside me from the very beginning. Tony has listened to more half-formed ideas, late-night brainstorms, and "*does this make sense*?" questions than any one person should reasonably endure.

To **Brian Kittrell**, coworker, friend, and fellow advocate for Veterans. Brian's passion for this community mirrors my own, and his creative eye helped bring this book's cover to life. I'm grateful for his support, his ideas, and his ability to say, "*Yeah, that'll work*," at exactly the right moment.

To the many **Veterans who reached out** after reading the first book — thank you. Your stories of clarity, hope, and finally beginning your own journey encouraged me more than you can imagine. Every message, every success, every "*I finally understand this*" reminded me why this work matters.

And finally, to the broader **Veteran community**, whose resilience and strength continue to encourage me daily. This book, like the one before it, exists because you deserve clarity, respect, and the benefits you earned through your service.

§ § § EXTRA INSIGHTS § § §

Before you close this book, I want to say something directly to you—not as an author, not as an advocate, but simply as one person to another. You chose to spend your time here, learning, questioning, and pushing for clarity in a system that doesn't always make things easy. That choice matters. It says something about your determination, your resilience, and your willingness to take ownership of your journey.

If anything in these pages helped you feel more confident, more informed, or even just a little less alone in the process, then I'm grateful. That's why I wrote this. You've carried more than most people will ever understand, and you deserve support that meets you with honesty and respect. Thank you for giving me the chance to walk alongside you for a few chapters of your story. Wherever you go from here, I hope you carry forward the reminder that your voice matters—and your benefits are worth fighting for.

§ § § § § § § § §

Appendix A: *Glossary of VA Terms*

You're not alone in this. Thousands of Veterans have walked this path — and you're about to walk it with clarity and confidence.

Aid & Attendance (A&A)
An additional pension benefit for Veterans or surviving spouses who need help with daily activities such as bathing, dressing, or mobility.

Appeal
A request for the VA to review a decision you disagree with.

At Least As Likely As Not
A medical phrase meaning a 50% or greater chance a condition is related to service — the magic words for service connection.

Asymptomatic
A medical term meaning you have a condition but no noticeable symptoms.

Benefit of the Doubt
If evidence is evenly balanced, the VA must side with the Veteran.

Buddy Statement
A written statement from someone who witnessed or can confirm your symptoms, events, or limitations.

Baseline Level of Disability
The level of disability *before* a condition was worsened by a service-connected condition (important for secondary claims).

C-File (*Claims File*)
Your complete VA record — claims, evidence, decisions, exams, everything.

C&P Exam (*Compensation & Pension Exam*)
A medical exam used to evaluate your condition for rating purposes.

Claim
A formal request for VA benefits.

Chronic
A condition that is long-lasting or recurring.

Compensation
Monthly tax-free payments for service-connected disabilities.

Countable Income
Your income minus certain deductions — especially medical expenses. The VA pension formula is basically "*income minus reality*."

Credible Evidence
Believable, consistent, and reliable — not necessarily perfect.

DBQ (*Disability Benefits Questionnaire*)
Standardized form used to document symptoms and limitations.

Decision Letter
VA's written explanation of your rating, effective date, and reasoning.

Direct Service Connection
A condition directly caused by military service.

Diagnostic Code (DC)
The VA's numerical code for rating specific conditions.

Duty to Assist
The VA's responsibility to help gather evidence for your claim.
They don't always get everything, but they do have to try.

Effective Date
The date the VA uses to determine when your benefits begin.

Evidence
Medical records, statements, exams, and documents used to support your claim.

Exacerbation
A flare-up or worsening of symptoms.

Functional Loss
How your condition affects your ability to work, move, think, or perform daily tasks.

Frequency, Severity, Duration
Three key factors the VA uses to evaluate symptoms.

HLR (*Higher-Level Review*)
A type of appeal where a senior reviewer re-examines your claim without new evidence.

Hypertension
High blood pressure — a common VA-rated condition.

Intent to File (ITF)
A simple form that locks in your effective date and gives you up to a year to submit your claim.

Impairment
A loss of function or ability.

Intent to File
a simple form that locks in your effective date and gives you up to a year to gather evidence.

Lay Evidence
Statements from you, family, or friends describing symptoms or events — no medical training required.

Limitation of Motion
Reduced ability to move a joint — a major factor in musculoskeletal ratings.

Medical Nexus
A medical opinion linking your condition to your service.

MST (*Military Sexual Trauma*)
Trauma resulting from sexual assault or harassment during service.

Maximum Medical Improvement (MMI)
The point where a condition is unlikely to improve further.

Nexus Letter
A written medical opinion explaining how your condition is connected to service.

Non-Service-Connected (NSC)
A condition not linked to military service.

Pension
A needs-based benefit for wartime Veterans with limited income and medical expenses.

Presumptive Condition
A condition the VA automatically assumes is service-connected based on specific exposures or service periods.

Primary Condition
A condition directly caused by service.

Rating Decision
The VA's official determination of your disability percentage.

Remand
When the Board sends your case back for more evidence or clarification.

Residuals
Ongoing symptoms or limitations that remain after an injury or illness.

Secondary Service Connection
A condition caused or worsened by a service-connected disability.

SMC (*Special Monthly Compensation*)
Additional compensation for specific circumstances like mobility issues, loss of use, or needing daily assistance.

Stabilized Rating
A rating that's been in place for several years and is less likely to be reduced. The longer you've had a rating, the more protection.

Stressor
A traumatic event used to support PTSD claims.

TDIU (*Total Disability Based on Individual Unemployability*)
A benefit that pays at the 100% rate if your service-connected conditions prevent you from working.

Trigger
Something that causes symptoms to flare — often used in mental health claims.

VA Math
The VA's unique method of combining disability ratings — it is percentages, so is "different".

VSO (*Veterans Service Officer*)
A trained advocate who helps file and manage claims for free.

Wartime Service
Service during specific periods defined by Congress — combat not required.

† † † † †

Every branch had its own language,
but we all understood one universal truth:

If the military could turn something simple into an acronym,
it absolutely would.
Half the time the jargon made no sense at all —
yet somehow, it brought us together,
and we always knew exactly what we meant.

† † † † †

Appendix B: *Primary & Secondary Conditions*

You don't need to understand everything today.
You just need to take the next step.

Understanding how the VA evaluates different medical conditions can feel like trying to read a map without a legend — the pieces are there, but the meaning isn't always obvious. This section breaks down the most common conditions Veterans file for and explains, in plain English, what the VA actually looks for when assigning ratings. No legal jargon, no medical maze — just clear guidance to help you see where your symptoms fit and what evidence strengthens your case.

Whether you're looking at primary conditions, secondary conditions, or the rating criteria themselves, remember this: the VA isn't just rating diagnoses — it's rating how those conditions shape your daily life. These cheat sheets are designed to help you connect the dots, understand the bigger picture, and make sure nothing important gets overlooked. Your health story is more than one condition, and you deserve a rating that reflects the reality you live with every day.

PTSD / Mental Health Conditions

The VA rates all mental health conditions using the same scale (0–100%). They look at:

- How often symptoms occur
- How severe they are
- How much they affect work, relationships, and daily life

Examples:

- 30% — Occasional decrease in work efficiency
- 50% — Reduced Reliability and Productivity
- 70% — Major impairment in most areas of life
- 100% — Total occupational and social impairment

Back & Neck Conditions

Ratings depend on:

- Range of motion
- Pain on movement
- Muscle spasms
- Functional loss
- Incapacitating episodes (*for disc issues*)

Examples:

- 10–20% — Limited motion with pain
- 40% — Severe limitation or forward flexion ≤ 30°
- 50–100% — Spinal fusion or ankylosis

Knee Conditions

The VA looks at:

- Flexion (*bending*)
- Extension (*straightening*)
- Instability
- Pain and functional loss

Examples:

- 10% — Painful motion
- 20–30% — Moderate to severe instability
- 40–50% — Severe limitation of extension

Migraines

Ratings depend on:

- Frequency
- Duration
- Severity
- Impact on ability to function

Examples:

- 30% — Monthly prostrating attacks
- 50% — Very frequent, completely prostrating attacks with severe economic impact

---

Sleep Apnea

Ratings depend on:

- Daytime sleepiness
- CPAP use
- Breathing issues

Examples:

- 30% — Persistent daytime sleepiness
- 50% — Requires CPAP
- 100% — Chronic respiratory failure

Tinnitus

- 10% max — Ringing in one or both ears

Hearing Loss

Ratings depend on:

- Audiology test results
- Speech discrimination scores

Hypertension

Ratings depend on blood pressure readings:

- 10% — Diastolic 100+ or systolic 160+
- 20–40% — Higher sustained readings

Scars

Rated based on:

- Pain
- Size
- Location
- Stability

Diabetes (*Type II*)

Ratings depend on:

- Medication
- Diet
- Activity restrictions
- Complications

Examples:

- 20% — Requires medication
- 40% — Requires insulin + restricted diet
- 60–100% — Severe complications

---

† † † † †

You can be rated for multiple conditions —
and even if each rating is small,
they can add up to meaningful monthly compensation.

† † † † †

About Secondary Conditions

Many Veterans don't realize that some of their most frustrating symptoms aren't separate issues at all — they're *secondary conditions* caused or worsened by something the VA has already acknowledged. This section helps you connect the dots. By understanding how one condition can lead to another, you can make sure your full health picture is recognized and rated fairly. Think of this as your roadmap to the "*hidden*" parts of your claim — the ones that often make the biggest difference.

Below are some of the most common — and most overlooked — secondary conditions. These examples don't cover everything, but they give you a strong starting point for spotting connections in your own health.

Orthopaedic Conditions → Secondary Issues

Primary issues like back, knee, ankle, or neck problems often lead to:

- Radiculopathy (*nerve pain down arms or legs*)
- Sciatica
- Hip or opposite-side knee pain (*from altered gait*)
- Foot problems (*plantar fasciitis, flat feet*)
- Migraines (*from neck issues*)
- Depression (*from chronic pain*)

PTSD / Anxiety / Depression → Secondary Issues

Mental health conditions frequently cause or worsen:

- Sleep apnea
- GERD / acid reflux
- Irritable bowel syndrome (IBS)
- Hypertension
- Migraines
- Alcohol or substance use disorders
- Erectile dysfunction

Sleep Apnea → Secondary Issues

Sleep apnea can contribute to:

- Hypertension
- Heart disease
- Daytime fatigue → accidents or injuries
- Depression or anxiety

Diabetes (Type II) → Secondary Issues

Diabetes often leads to:

- Peripheral neuropathy
- Kidney disease
- Vision problems
- Erectile dysfunction
- Skin conditions
- Cardiovascular issues

Tinnitus / Hearing Loss → Secondary Issues

These can contribute to:

- Anxiety
- Depression
- Sleep disturbances
- Concentration problems

GERD / Digestive Issues → Secondary Issues

Often linked to:

- Dental erosion
- Sleep disturbances
- Anxiety
- Chronic cough

Medication Side Effects → Secondary Issues

Many medications used for service-connected conditions can cause:

- Weight gain
- Liver issues
- Kidney issues
- Sexual dysfunction
- Sleep problems
- Digestive issues

Traumatic Brain Injury (TBI) → Secondary Issues

TBI can lead to:

- Migraines
- Memory problems
- Mood disorders
- Sleep disorders
- Hormonal issues
- Vision problems

Chronic Pain → Secondary Issues

Long-term pain often causes:

- Depression
- Anxiety
- Sleep problems
- Fatigue
- Mobility issues → new joint problems

Heart Conditions → Secondary Issues

Heart disease can lead to:

- Kidney issues
- Fatigue
- Shortness of breath
- Depression

Appendix C: *Important Contacts*

You can request your military personnel file (OMPF)
from the National Archives —
and it often contains evaluations, training records,
and incident reports you forgot existed.

Navigating the complexities of veteran benefits and support systems can be overwhelming—especially when time, clarity, and access are critical. This appendix provides a curated list of trusted contacts and organizations that serve veterans and their families across a range of needs, from healthcare and education to legal assistance and crisis support.

While every effort has been made to ensure the accuracy and relevance of the information provided, organizations and services may change over time. For that reason, we encourage you to verify details directly with each resource to ensure you receive the most current and effective support available.

American Job Center (*Veterans*)

No-cost career counseling, job search assistance, and veteran-focused hiring events

Web: **https://www.careeronestop.org/Veterans/default.aspx**

Phone: 1-877-872-5627 (1-877-US2-JOBS)

Beneficiary Travel Program

Reimbursement for travel to VA medical appointments

Web: **https://www.va.gov/health-care/file-travel-pay-reimbursement/**

Phone: 1-800-949-1000

Caregiver Support Program (PCAFC)

Stipends, training, counseling, and respite services for family caregivers of seriously injured veterans

Web: **https://www.caregiver.va.gov/**

Phone: 1-855-260-3274

Commemorative Plaque and Urn Benefit:

Survivors of eligible veterans can apply for and receive a commemorative plaque and urn for their veteran.

Web: **https://www.va.gov/burials-memorials/memorial-items/headstones-markers-medallions/**

Phone: 1- 800-697-6947

---

eBenefits

Self-service site to apply for and track VA/DoD benefits, appeals, and claims status (ID.me required)

Web: **https://www.ebenefits.va.gov/**

Phone: 1-800-983-0937

GI Bill® Education Benefits

Apply for and manage Post-9/11, Montgomery, or Survivors' GI Bill benefits; compare schools and certify enrollment

Web: **https://www.va.gov/education/**

Phone: 1-888-442-4551 (1-888-GIBILL1)

ID.me

Secure digital identity-verification service to confirm veteran status online

Web: **https://www.id.me/**

Phone: 1-888-454-9366

Military OneSource

24/7 DoD-sponsored support for counseling, financial guidance, relocation, and family services

Web: **https://www.militaryonesource.mil/**

Phone: 1-800-342-9647

National Call Center for Homeless Veterans

24/7 confidential assistance to prevent or exit veteran homelessness

Web: **https://www.va.gov/homeless/national-call-center.asp**

Phone: 1-877-424-3838 (1-877-4AID-VET)

National Cemetery Scheduling Office

Arrange burial in national cemeteries, headstones, markers, and full military funeral honors

Web: **https://www.va.gov/burials-memorials/schedule-a-burial/**

Phone: 1-800-535-1117

National Resource Directory

Centralized directory of vetted support services for veterans, caregivers, and families

Web: **https://nrd.gov/**

Office of General Counsel Accreditation Search

Lookup accredited VSOs, Claims Agents, and attorneys authorized to represent claimants before the VA

Web: **https://www.va.gov/ogc/apps/accreditation/index.asp**

SAM.gov

Register your business for federal contracts; obtain a Unique Entity Identifier (UEI)

Web: **https://sam.gov/**

Phone: 1-866-606-8220 (Federal Service Desk)

U.S. Court of Appeals for Veterans Claims Clerk's Office

Filing appeals after Board decisions

Web: **http://www.uscourts.cavc.gov/**

Phone: 202-501-5970

VA.GOV

Official U.S. Department of Veterans Affairs portal for benefits, health care, and resources

Web: **https://www.va.gov/**

Phone: 1-800-827-1000

VA Adaptive Sports Program

Grants to cover equipment, coaching, and travel for veterans in adaptive sports

Web: **https://department.va.gov/veteran-sports/**

Phone: 1-800-749-8387

VA Dental Insurance Program (VADIP)

Voluntary, low-cost dental plans for enrolled veterans and their families

Web: **https://www.va.gov/health-care/about-va-health-benefits/dental-care/dental-insurance/**

Phone: 1-877-222-8387 (1-877-222-VETS)

VA Foreign Medical Program (FMP)

Reimbursement for approved service-connected care received overseas

Web: **https://www.va.gov/communitycare/programs/veterans/fmp/index.asp**

Phone: 1-877-345-8179

VA Home Loan Program

Information on eligibility, entitlement, and application for VA-backed mortgage loans

Web: **https://www.benefits.va.gov/homeloans/**

Phone: 1-877-827-3702

VA Homeless Veteran Reintegration Program (HVRP)

Job placement and training for homeless vets

Web: **https://www.dol.gov/agencies/vets/programs/hvrp**

Phone: 1-877-424-3838

VA Telehealth Services Help Desk

Technical support for video and home-based care

Web: **https://telehealth.va.gov/help-center**

Phone: 1-877-741-3400

VA Vet Center Call Center

Confidential readjustment counseling and outreach

Web: **https://www.vetcenter.va.gov/**

Phone: 1-877-927-8387

VetCert (MySBA Certifications)

Portal to apply for Veteran-Owned (VOSB) and Service-Disabled VOSB certifications

Web: **https://veterans.certify.sba.gov/**

Phone: 1-800-827-5722

Veterans Benefits Administration

Manages disability compensation, pension, education, home-loan, and burial programs

Web: **https://benefits.va.gov/benefits/**

Phone: 1-800-827-1000

Veterans Business Outreach Center (VBOC) Locator

Find no-cost entrepreneurial mentoring, workshops, and SBA resource partners near you

Web: **https://www.sba.gov/local-assistance/resource-partners/veterans-business-outreach-center-vboc**

Phone: 1-800-827-5722

Veterans Crisis Line

24/7 crisis support—call 988 then press 1, text 838255, or chat online

Web: **https://www.veteranscrisisline.net/**

VetSuccess on Campus

VA career counseling and vocational-rehabilitation services located at colleges and universities

Web: **https://www.va.gov/careers-employment/vocational-rehabilitation/**

Phone: 1-800-827-1000

VET TEC Program

Technology-training vouchers (coding, cybersecurity) that don't exhaust GI Bill entitlement

Web: **https://www.va.gov/education/about-gi-bill-benefits/how-to-use-benefits/vettec-program/**

Phone: 1-888-442-4551

Vocational Rehabilitation & Employment (VR&E)

Job training, education planning, and employment services for veterans with service-connected disabilities

Web: **https://www.benefits.va.gov/vocrehab/**

Phone: 1-800-827-1000

Women Veterans Program Coordinator (National Office)

Gender-specific health care coordination

Web: **https://www.va.gov/womenvet/**

Phone: 1-855-829-6636

Yellow Ribbon Program

Tuition-gap funding for Post-9/11 GI Bill users at private or out-of-state institutions

Web: **https://www.va.gov/education/about-gi-bill-benefits/post-9-11/yellow-ribbon-program/**

Phone: 1-888-442-4551

---

§ § § EXTRA INSIGHTS § § §

Having the right phone numbers and websites is only half the battle—knowing how to use them is where the real power lies. Every VA office, hotline, and program has its own rhythm, its own strengths, and its own way of helping Veterans. When you reach out, you're not just calling an agency; you're connecting with people who handle these questions every day and know exactly how to point you in the right direction.

BEHIND THE CURTAIN: *Many VA representatives have access to internal notes, timelines, and status updates that Veterans never see on their own. A quick call can reveal where your claim is in the process, what evidence might still be needed, or whether something is waiting on a simple correction. Don't hesitate to use these contacts—they're part of the system you earned through your service, and they exist to help you move forward with clarity and confidence.*

§ § § § § § § § §

Appendix D: *C & P* *Exam Guidance*

Using short, vague statements like "my back hurts."
The VA needs specifics — when it started, how it affects you,
and what makes it worse.

Step-by-Step C&P exam guide

Before the exam

- Know what the exam is for.
- Check your claim: Look at which conditions you filed for so you know what the examiner will focus on.
- Review your symptoms. Think in terms of:
  - Frequency: How often?
  - Severity: How bad?
  - Impact: What does it stop you from doing?
- Make a simple list and write down:
  - Your main symptoms
  - When they started
  - How they affect work, sleep, relationships, and daily tasks
- Bring what you need, such as:
  - Glasses, hearing aids, mobility devices
  - A short symptom list
  - A caregiver or spouse (*if allowed*) who sees your daily struggles

---

During the exam

- Be honest, not heroic. This is not the time to "*tough it out.*"
- Describe how you are on your worst or average days, not your best days.
- Answer the question asked clearly and directly.
  - If they ask, "*How far can you walk?*" don't say "*I'm fine.*" Say, "*About half a block before the pain makes me stop.*"
- Describe impact, not just pain. Instead of "*My back hurts,*" say:
  - "*I can't stand more than 10 minutes.*"
  - "*I need help putting on my shoes.*"
  - "*I miss work when it flares.*"
- Correct misunderstandings politely.
- If the examiner says something that isn't accurate, you can say:
  - "*That's not quite right—what I meant was...*"

After the exam

- Write down what happened. As soon as you get home, jot down:
  - How long did the exam last
  - What was asked
  - What tests were done
  - Anything that felt off or incomplete
- Don't panic if it felt "*too quick.*" Many C&P exams are brief. A short exam doesn't automatically mean a bad result.
- Watch for follow-up. The exam report becomes evidence in your claim. If the decision doesn't match your reality, your notes can help with an appeal or supplemental claim.

Myth vs. Reality: C&P Exams

Myth: "*The examiner decides my rating.*"

Reality: The examiner only records information. The VA rater makes the decision using your records, your statements, and the exam report.

Myth: "*If the exam is short, I'm getting denied.*"

Reality: Many exams are brief. Length has nothing to do with outcome — clarity and documentation do.

Myth: "*I should act tough so I don't seem dramatic.*"

Reality: This is the one place where minimizing hurts you. Be honest about your worst and average days, not your best.

Myth: "*If the examiner is rude or cold, my claim is doomed.*"

Reality: Personality doesn't affect ratings. What matters is what's written in the report — and you can challenge inaccuracies later.

Myth: "*I can't bring notes.*"

Reality: You absolutely can. Notes help you stay focused and ensure you don't forget key symptoms.

Day-Of C&P Exam Checklist

Before You Leave Home

- Review your symptom list (*frequency, severity, impact*).
- Bring glasses, hearing aids, braces, canes, CPAP, or anything you use daily.
- Take medications as you normally would — don't change your routine.
- If allowed, bring a spouse or caregiver who sees your daily struggles.
- Remember: This is not a treatment appointment. It's documentation.

During the Exam

- Be honest, not heroic.
- Describe limitations, not just pain ("*I can't stand longer than 10 minutes*").
- If asked about a "*good day,*" explain how rare those are.
- If something hurts, say so — don't push through it.
- If the examiner misunderstands, politely correct them: "*Let me clarify — what I meant was...*"

After the Exam

- Write down what happened:
  - How long it lasted
  - What tests were done
  - Anything unusual
- Don't panic if it felt rushed — that's common.
- Watch for VA letters or requests for more information.
- If the decision doesn't match your reality, your notes help with appeals.

C&P Exam Red Flags — What to Watch For

These are moments during a C&P exam that should make a Veteran pause, take note, and document what happened afterward. They don't automatically mean the exam was "*bad,*" but they *do* mean the Veteran should pay closer attention to the final decision.

Red Flags During the Exam

- The examiner doesn't let you speak or cuts you off repeatedly. Your voice matters — the exam should reflect *your* experience.
- The examiner never asks about your worst days. VA ratings are based on average or typical functioning, not rare good days.
- The examiner doesn't review your records or seems unaware of your history. They should at least skim your file or ask clarifying questions.
- The exam feels rushed (*under 5 minutes*) with no meaningful questions. Short exams happen, but they should still be thorough.
- The examiner dismisses or minimizes your symptoms. "*That doesn't sound bad*" is not a medical evaluation.
- The examiner performs physical tests incorrectly or unsafely. Especially for back, knee, or neck exams.
- You're asked to do movements that cause sharp pain and aren't allowed to stop. You should never be pushed beyond safe limits.
- The examiner seems confused about the purpose of the exam. (*Yes, this happens more than people think.*)
- Even if you think it is going bad, stay calm and finish the exam.

C&P Exam Do's and Don'ts

Do's

Do be honest about your worst and average days.

The VA rates limitations, not toughness.

Do describe impact, not just pain.

Say what the condition *stops you from doing.*

Do bring your assistive devices.

If you use it at home, bring it to the exam.

Do take your medications as usual.

The VA needs to see your real, daily baseline.

Do correct misunderstandings politely.

"Let me clarify — what I meant was..."

Do stay calm and focused.

You're there to document, not to impress.

Do write down what happened afterward.

Your notes can help if the exam report is inaccurate.

Don'ts

Don't minimize your symptoms.

This is not the time to "*push through it.*"

Don't guess or make up answers.

If you don't know, say so.

Don't let the examiner rush you.

You deserve time to explain your symptoms clearly.

Don't perform movements that cause sharp pain.

Stop immediately and say, "*That hurts too much.*"

Don't assume the examiner decides your rating.

They only document — the VA rater decides.

Don't panic if the exam is short.

Short exams are common and not a bad sign.

What To Do If Your C&P Exam Was Bad

Step 1: *Write Down Everything Immediately*

Include:

- What the examiner asked
- What they didn't ask
- How long the exam lasted
- Any concerning behavior
- Any tests that weren't performed correctly

Your memory is sharpest right after the exam.

Step 2: *Request a Copy of Your C&P Exam Report*

You can view it in:

- VA.gov (*often appears within days*)
- Your VA medical records
- Your C-File (*if needed*)

Reading the report helps you see whether your symptoms were accurately documented.

Step 3: *Compare the Report to Your Reality*

Ask yourself:

- Did the examiner record what you actually said?
- Did they leave out major symptoms?
- Did they misstate your abilities?
- Did they claim you denied symptoms you actually reported?

If something is wrong, don't panic — it can be fixed.

Step 4: ***Gather Supporting Evidence***

If the report is inaccurate, consider adding:

- A personal statement clarifying what happened
- A buddy or caregiver statement
- Updated private medical records
- A DBQ from your own doctor (*if available*)

Step 5: ***File a Supplemental Claim or Appeal (If needed)***

If the decision is based on a flawed exam, you can:

- Submit a Supplemental Claim with new evidence
- Request a Higher-Level Review (HLR)
- Appeal directly to the Board of Veterans' Appeals

Your notes and evidence become the backbone of your challenge.

Step 6: ***Remember — One Bad Exam Does not Define Your Claim***

Veterans win appeals every day because they documented what went wrong. The system isn't perfect, but it *is* fixable.

---

† † † † †

You can request a copy of your entire VA claims file (C-File).
It's a powerful tool for understanding
your history and planning future steps.

† † † † †

How to Describe Your Symptoms

This guide teaches Veterans how to communicate clearly and effectively — something most struggle with during C&P exams.

Use the VA's Three Magic Words

The VA evaluates symptoms based on:

- Frequency — How often does it happen?
- Severity — How bad is it?
- Duration — How long does it last?

Example:
"Three to four times a week, the pain becomes so severe I have to lie down for an hour."

Focus on Functional Impact

Instead of saying:

- *"My back hurts."*

Say:

- *"I can't stand longer than 10 minutes."*
- *"I need help putting on socks and shoes."*
- *"I miss work when it flares."*

The VA rates limitations, not diagnoses.

Describe Your Worst and Average Days

Not your rare, good days.

Example:
"On an average day, I can walk half a block before stopping. On a bad day, I can't leave the house."

Be Specific, Not Vague

Instead of:

- *"Sometimes it bothers me."*

Say:

- *"Four to five days a week, the pain wakes me up at night."*

Explain Triggers and Consequences

- What makes it worse?
- What happens afterward?
- How long does recovery take?

Example:
"If I lift anything over 10 pounds, I'm in pain for the rest of the day."

Do not Downplay or Overstate

Just be accurate. Your goal is clarity, not drama.

Use Real-Life Examples

These help the examiner understand your daily reality.

Example:
"I can't sit through a 30-minute meeting without shifting constantly or standing up."

---

§ § § EXTRA INSIGHTS § § §

A C&P exam can feel like the most stressful part of the entire claims process, but here's something worth remembering: the exam isn't a test of toughness or memory—it's a chance to tell your story plainly and honestly. You don't have to perform, impress, or convince. You just have to be real about what life looks like on your hardest days.

<u>INSIDER TIP</u>: *Most examiners rely heavily on the details you provide in the moment. When you describe your symptoms clearly, give examples, and avoid minimizing what you're going through, you're giving the examiner exactly what they need to document your condition accurately. A calm, truthful conversation often does more for your claim than any stack of paperwork.*

§ § § § § § § §

Appendix E: *Benefits by Disability Rating*

Identifying even one overlooked condition
— primary or secondary —
can significantly change your overall rating
and monthly compensation.

This appendix gives a clear breakdown of the benefits veterans and their families may be eligible for at each VA disability rating. **VA rules may change** , so treat this appendix as a succinct starting point to orient yourself. Always verify!

0% Compensable (*TWO or more 0% MAY be compensated at 10% Rate*)

- No Cost Health Care and Prescription Drugs for Service-Connected Disabilities (*if income limits are met)*
- Travel Pay for Healthcare Appointments for Service-Connected Conditions
- Exchange/Commissary/MWR Access Privileges
- VA Life insurance guaranteed acceptance up to $40,000
- VADIP (*VA Dental Insurance*) if Enrolled in VA Healthcare
- Non-VA Urgent Care visits at $30/visit including 14-day prescription (*Priority Group 6*)
    - $0 for Service-Connected Conditions
    - $30 for Non-Service-Connected Conditions
    - Includes 14-day Prescriptions
- Non-VA Emergency Room care
    - Must notify VA within 72 hours:
        - Email: **VHAEmergencyNotification@va.gov**
        - Call 844-72HRVHA (844-724-7842)
- Waiver of VA Home Loan Funding Fee
- Check the Federal Benefits Matrix, State-Specific Benefits, and Your State VA Website

http://go.VeteranRollCall.org/matrix

0% Non-Compensable Rating Benefits Include:

- No Cost Health Care and Prescription Drugs for Service-Connected Disabilities (*if income limits are me)*
- Travel Pay for Healthcare Appointments for Service-Connected Conditions
- Exchange/Commissary/MWR Access Privileges
- VA Life insurance guaranteed acceptance up to $40,000
- VADIP (*VA Dental Insurance*) if enrolled in VA Healthcare
- 3 No Charge Non-VA Urgent Care visits (*Priority Group 5*)
    - Includes 14-day Prescriptions
- Non-VA Emergency Room care
    - Must notify VA within 72 hours:
        - Email: **VHAEmergencyNotification@va.gov**
        - Call 844-72HRVHA (844-724-7842)
- Check the Federal Benefits Matrix, State-Specific Benefits, and Your State VA Website

http://go.VeteranRollCall.org/matrix

10%-20% Rating Benefits Include:

- Monthly Tax-Free Financial Compensation
- Full Healthcare with Some Copays *for Non-Service-Connected Conditions*
- Travel Pay for Healthcare Appointments *for Service-Connected Conditions*
- Waiver of VA Home Loan Funding Fee
- Veteran Readiness & Employment (VR&E) at 20% or More
    - *10% with a Serious Employment Handicap*
    - *May also Include VA Dental*
- Exchange/Commissary/MWR Access Privileges
- Possible Social Security Disability Insurance (SSDI) Concurrent Benefits
- VA Life insurance guaranteed acceptance up to $40,000
- VADIP (*VA Dental Insurance Program*) for Veterans Enrolled in VA Healthcare
- 3 No-Charge non-VA Urgent Care Visits Per Calendar Year (*Priority Group 3*)
- Non-VA Emergency Room care
    - Must notify VA within 72 hours:
        - Email: **VHAEmergencyNotification@va.gov**
        - Call 844-72HRVHA (844-724-7842)
- Hearing Aids and Eye Exams and Glasses are Included with VA Healthcare
- You May Be Reviewed in the Future – Keep Doctors Informed of Rated Conditions
- Also Check the Federal Benefits Matrix:

  http://go.VeteranRollCall.org/matrix
- Your State Also Has Benefits Which May Include Tax Exemptions, Tuition Waivers, etc.

30%-40% Rating Benefits Include:

- Monthly Tax-Free Financial Compensation
- Full Healthcare with Some Copays for Non-Service-Connected Conditions
- Travel Pay for Healthcare Appointments
- Additional Monthly Compensation for Spouse/Dependents
- Waiver of VA Home Loan Funding Fee
- Veteran Readiness & Employment (VR&E)
  - *May also include VA Dental*
- Exchange/Commissary/MWR Access Privileges
- Possible Social Security Disability Insurance (SSDI) Concurrent Benefits
- VA Life insurance guaranteed acceptance up to $40,000
- VADIP (*VA Dental Insurance Program*) for Veterans Enrolled in VA Healthcare
- 3 No-Charge non-VA Urgent Care Visits Per Calendar Year (*Priority Group 2*)
- Non-VA Emergency Room care
  - Must notify VA within 72 hours:
    - Email: **VHAEmergencyNotification@va.gov**
    - Call 844-72HRVHA (844-724-7842)
- Hearing Aids and Eye Exams and Glasses are Included with VA Healthcare
- You May Be Reviewed in the Future – Keep Doctors Informed of Rated Conditions
- Also Check the Federal Benefits Matrix:

  http://go.VeteranRollCall.org/matrix
- Your State Also Has Benefits Which May Include Tax Exemptions, Tuition Waivers, etc.

† † † † †

VA disability compensation isn't just about the veteran.
It protects the family too. Certain ratings unlock benefits like
education support for dependents, health coverage,
and survivor compensation.
Always check how your rating impacts those you love.

† † † † †

50%-90% Rating Benefits Include:

- Monthly Tax-Free Financial Compensation
- Full Healthcare with NO Copays
- Travel Pay for Healthcare Appointments
- Additional Monthly Compensation for Spouse/Dependents
- Waiver of VA Home Loan Funding Fee
- Veteran Readiness & Employment (VR&E)
    - *May also include VA Dental*
- Exchange/Commissary/MWR Access Privileges
- Possible Social Security Disability Insurance (SSDI) Concurrent Benefits
- VA Life insurance guaranteed acceptance up to $40,000
- VADIP (*VA Dental Insurance Program*) for Veterans Enrolled in VA Healthcare
- 3 No-Charge non-VA Urgent Care Visits Per Calendar Year (*Priority Group 1*)
- Non-VA Emergency Room care
    - Must notify VA within 72 hours:
        - Email: **VHAEmergencyNotification@va.gov**
        - Call 844-72HRVHA (844-724-7842)
- Hearing Aids and Eye Exams and Glasses are Included with VA Healthcare
- You May Be Reviewed in the Future – Keep Doctors Informed of Rated Conditions
- Also Check the Federal Benefits Matrix:

  http://go.VeteranRollCall.org/matrix
- Your State Also Has Benefits Which May Include Tax Exemptions, Tuition Waivers, etc.

<u>100% TDIU *(Total Disability – Individual Unemployability)* Benefits Include:</u>

- Monthly Tax-Free Financial Compensation
- At 100% TDIU You Have Restrictions on Income from Employment
- **Additional If You Are Also Permanent & Total (*P&T*)**
    - CHAMPVA (*dependent medical)*
    - VADIP (*VA Dental Insurance Program*) for dependent's if CHAMPVA eligible
    - Chapter 35 DEA (*dependent's education*)
    - Federal student loan forgiveness
- Space-A Flights (*Cat VI*) - Veteran and Eligible Dependents
- Department of Defense (DoD) ID card
- VA Life insurance guaranteed acceptance up to $40,000
- Full Healthcare with NO Copays
- No-Cost Dental Care for Veterans Enrolled in VA healthcare
- Travel Pay for Healthcare Appointments
- Additional Monthly Compensation for Spouse/Dependents
- Waiver of VA Home Loan Funding Fee
- Veteran Readiness & Employment (VR&E)
- Exchange/Commissary/MWR Access Privileges
- Possible Social Security Disability Insurance (SSDI) Concurrent Benefits
- 3 No-Charge non-VA Urgent Care Visits Per Calendar Year (*Priority Group 1*)

- Non-VA Emergency Room care
  - Must notify VA within 72 hours:
    - Email: **VHAEmergencyNotification@va.gov**
    - Call 844-72HRVHA (844-724-7842)
- Hearing Aids and Eye Exams and Glasses are Included with VA Healthcare
- You May Be Reviewed in the Future – Keep Doctors Informed of Rated Conditions
  - *If P&T, typically WILL NOT have review examinations*
- Also Check the Federal Benefits Matrix:

  http://go.VeteranRollCall.org/matrix
- Your State Also Has Benefits Which May Include Tax Exemptions, Tuition Waivers, etc.

100% *Single or Combined Totaling 100%* Rating Benefits Include:

- Monthly Tax-Free Financial Compensation
- At 100% Schedular, You Can Work with No Restrictions
- **Additional if you are also Permanent & Total (*P&T*)**
    - CHAMPVA (*dependent medical*)
    - VADIP (*VA Dental Insurance Program*) for Dependent's if CHAMPVA Eligible
    - Chapter 35 DEA (*Dependent's Education*)
    - Federal Student Loan Forgiveness
- Space-A Flights (*Cat VI*) - Veteran and Eligible Dependents
- Department of Defense (DoD) ID Card
- VA Life insurance guaranteed acceptance up to $40,000
- Full Healthcare with NO Copays
- No-Cost Dental Care for Veterans Enrolled in VA healthcare
- Travel Pay for Healthcare Appointments
- Additional Monthly Compensation for Spouse/Dependents
- Waiver of VA Home Loan Funding Fee
- Veteran Readiness & Employment (VR&E)
- Exchange/Commissary/MWR Access Privileges
- Possible Social Security Disability Insurance (SSDI) Concurrent Benefits
- 3 No-Charge non-VA Urgent Care Visits Per Calendar Year (*Priority Group 1*)

- Non-VA Emergency Room care
    - Must notify VA within 72 hours:
        - Email: **VHAEmergencyNotification@va.gov**
        - Call 844-72HRVHA (844-724-7842)
- Hearing Aids and Eye Exams and Glasses are Included with VA Healthcare
- You May Be Reviewed in the Future – Keep Doctors Informed of Rated Conditions
    - *If P&T, typically WILL NOT have review examinations*
- Also Check the Federal Benefits Matrix:

  http://go.VeteranRollCall.org/matrix
- Your State Also Has Benefits Which May Include Tax Exemptions, Tuition Waivers, etc.

---

§ § § EXTRA INSIGHTS § § §

Seeing your benefits laid out by disability percentage can be eye-opening, but here's something most Veterans never hear: your rating isn't just a number—it's a doorway. Each increase unlocks new programs, new forms of support, and new opportunities that weren't available before. The VA designed these thresholds intentionally, and knowing what opens at each level helps you plan your next steps with confidence rather than guesswork.

<u>BEHIND THE CURTAIN</u>: *Many Veterans don't realize that VA staff use the same benefit matrix you just reviewed. When your rating changes, internal systems automatically flag new entitlements you may qualify for—but they don't always notify you. That's why understanding your benefits at each percentage is so powerful. It puts you in the driver's seat, ensuring you never miss a resource you've earned simply because no one mentioned it.*

§ § § § § § § § §

The 5-10-20 Rules

These describe how protection for VA disability ratings increases the longer a veteran's award remains unchanged. These rules add layers of protection the longer a veteran's award stands, but they do not create absolute immunity—fraud and CUE (*Clear and Unmistakable Error*) remain exception pathways for the VA to make rating adjustments. It is important to remember these protections apply to continuous ratings/service connections. Temporary ratings or staged ratings may not qualify

The 5-Year Rule: After a disability rating has remained at the same level for 5 continuous years, that rating becomes effectively "*stabilized.*" To reduce the rating the VA must show sustained improvement in the veteran's condition under ordinary conditions of life—not just a temporary or equivocal change.

The 10-Year Rule: If service connection (*the finding that a condition is service-connected*) has existed for 10 or more years, the VA may not sever service connection except in cases of fraud or clear and unmistakable error (CUE) in the original award.

The 20-Year Rule: Ratings or service connections that have remained unchanged for 20 years enjoy the most protection. After 20 years the VA generally may not reduce a rating unless there is evidence the original award was obtained by fraud or the record contains a clear and unmistakable error.

MYTH:

"My story doesn't matter — the VA only cares about paperwork."

REALITY:

Your story is evidence.

Clear, honest statements often fill the gaps that records can't.

About the Author

Wiltz Cutrer is an Accredited VA Claims Agent, educator, and advocate whose mission is simple: help Veterans understand the benefits they earned through service. After more than three decades working in information technology—where he learned that clarity can turn confusion into confidence—he now focuses his time on outreach, education, and guiding Veterans through the often-overwhelming VA benefits and programs.

Growing up as a Coast Guard dependent, Wiltz spent his childhood moving up and down the East Coast before enlisting in the U.S. Navy just two weeks after high school graduation. He served as a Cryptologic Technician–Maintenance (CTM) and carries the perspective of a disabled Veteran into every aspect of his work.

His advocacy began informally on the shop floor at Nucor, where he shared benefit insights with teammates. Those conversations grew into VeteranRollCall.org, a resource hub dedicated to helping Veterans and families make sense of their benefits. That mission expanded into seminars, community outreach, and the Veteran Roll Call Series—beginning with *Making Sense of What You've Earned.*

Wiltz is also the author of two technology guides, *Don't Throw IT—Get to Know IT* and *I Turned IT On—Now What?*, where his hallmark remains the same: clear language, real-world examples, and a genuine desire to empower.

At home, Wiltz enjoys life with his wife, Kristen, and their children, Wiltz III and Izabella—along with a few beloved dogs and cats who run the household with more authority than anyone admits. He treasures family game nights, weekend fishing trips, morning lattes, and planning magical Walt Disney World getaways as a Disney planner.

Your story isn't finished.

The next chapter is yours to write as you move forward.

Made in the USA
Monee, IL
04 November 2026

67383151R00144